WHITMER'S GUIDE TO TOTAL WELLNESS

WHITMER'S GUIDE TO TOTAL WELLNESS

Visualization Techniques for a Better, Healthier, and Longer Life

By R. WILLIAM WHITMER

DIRECTOR, WELLNESS CENTERS OF AMERICA

Drawings by Esther Lee

DOUBLEDAY & COMPANY, INC., GARDEN CITY, NEW YORK

1982

Library of Congress Cataloging in Publication Data

Whitmer, R. William, 1934–
Whitmer's Guide to Total Wellness.

1. Health. 2. Health behavior. 3. Behavior modification.
4. Visualization. I. Title. II. Title: Guide to total wellness.
RA776.W53 613

AACR2

ISBN: 0-385-17556-6
Library of Congress Catalog Card Number 81–43113

Printed in the United States of America

First Edition

This book is dedicated to my father
Roy William Whitmer
who gave so much and took so little

CONTENTS

ILLUSTRATIONS

ACKNOWLEDGMENTS

I am forever grateful and thankful to several individuals who have made major contributions not only to this book, but also to the establishment of this wellness concept. I want to thank Dr. John Burrett for his continuous encouragement, advice, and friendship. Charles Roe, Bill Jorden, Jay Johnston, Ralph Fuentes, and Wayne Nellums each made significant contributions.

I want to extend my appreciation to Judy Sargent and Suzanne Richardson for transforming the endless numbers of handwritten pages into a neat and well-organized manuscript. I am grateful to Esther Lee, an artist of extraordinary talent who was able to convert my words and concepts into pictures.

My editor, Barry Lippman, deserves special recognition. His editorial comments and suggestions have added immeasurably to the book. My agent, Richard Pine, provided encouragement from the first time we discussed the concept of this book and has constantly given me greatly appreciated counsel.

Most importantly, I want to thank my wife, Mary Frances, and sons, Bill and John, for tolerating my erratic hours while the book was being written and my extensive travel schedule.

R.W.W.

FOREWORD

This is an important, easily readable, and timely book. Every family in the United States would benefit by reading it.

This book is about our health and what we, as individuals, can do to improve it and live longer, happier, and disease-free lives. It tells us how we sometimes unknowingly ruin our health gradually over many years and what we can do about reversing this by discarding bad health habits. This book is full of good, sensible, and practical advice on how to change your lifestyle so as to minimize your chances of being disabled or dying from something which, with a little more care, might be prevented.

The leading causes of death in the United States are heart diseases, cancer, stroke, and lung diseases. Bill Whitmer in his lucid and easy-to-read style tells us how cigarettes, obesity, stress, lack of regular exercise, alcohol, salt, caffeine, and other factors often lead to these diseases, to disability, and to premature death. He shows us how to eliminate these poor health habits.

Whitmer's Guide to Total Wellness is an accurate portrait of what we know and what we don't know in the health sciences in the 1980s. If this book strikes your imagination and you decide to do something about your health—which I suspect you will—then start today and don't put it off until tomorrow. If there are things in it you don't understand and are concerned about, then discuss them with your family physician.

We in the United States enjoy a prosperity which no people in the history of the world have ever enjoyed in so much abundance. However, with this abundance comes subtle health risks which a lot of us are not fully aware of or choose to ignore. Bill Whitmer tells us how to enjoy this abundance and get more out of our lives.

He is to be congratulated on making an important contribution to good health in America.

JOHN K. VYDEN, M.D., F.A.C.C.
MEDICAL DIRECTOR
VASCULAR DIAGNOSTIC LABORATORY
AND CARDIAC REHABILITATION
CEDARS-SINAI MEDICAL CENTER
ASSOCIATE PROFESSOR OF MEDICINE
U.C.L.A. SCHOOL OF MEDICINE

Los Angeles, California
June 1981

INTRODUCTION

Are you strolling leisurely down the road to premature death? Probably so. Every year hundreds of thousands of Americans kill themselves by the lifestyle they lead. At last, many individuals are beginning to realize that personal lifestyle has a tremendous influence on the number of years they are going to live. In addition, attention is being given to the fact that lifestyle is the most important factor in establishing the quality of life, or how good or bad you feel.

The lifestyle you choose determines the degree of wellness you can expect. What is wellness? First, wellness goes far beyond the absence of illness. Wellness is a lifestyle, an attitude that enables a person to achieve his or her highest state of well-being. Wellness is feeling better and living longer.

I want to commend you for reading this book. It will have a profound impact on your life. In addition to adding extra years to your life, you will be instructed on how to enhance the quality of each extra day, month, and year you live. This book will help you make the most important discovery of your lifetime—*that you, all by yourself, can truly manipulate, influence, and alter your life-span. You are the master of your own fate in regard to adding to or subtracting from your life-span and quality of life.*

Lately, people have begun to examine our present health care system. Ninety percent of our health care money, time, talent, and resources are directed toward the treatment and cure of the various states of ill health. We have the best treatment services in the world. But the basic question is: "Why can't we do more to keep the population well?"

Because of this question, the Wellness Renaissance has started. The decades of the 1980s and 1990s will be unprecedented in consumer demand for services, programs, and facilities to help people stay well. Well—and out of the hospital. Well—and out of the doctor's office. Well—and on the job. Well—and feeling better and living longer.

Numerous medically oriented self-help books have been popular during the last few years. They teach you how to lose weight, get into better physical condition, cope with stress, consume a more nutritious diet, and much more. The majority of these books are fine. But this book is different in that it addresses the ultimate in medical self-help—how to feel better and live longer.

Is anything more important than life itself? It seems we rarely stop to reflect on this. We take life for granted, with no thought to how long we will live. We seem to believe that we automatically live for a predetermined number of years and that lifestyle or other external influences have no bearing on longevity or the quality of life. This is untrue.

The length of time you are going to live and the way you feel are directly related to how you treat your body. Abuse and misuse of the body results in acute and chronic disease, premature aging and premature death. The body will always respond to dedicated care. It will function better, with fewer problems and for a longer time.

Most people recognize the fact that smoking, everyday stress, obesity, poor nutrition, lack of regular exercise, and excessive consumption of alcohol are, in some way, harmful. So, why is it that tens of millions consciously and knowingly indulge in a lifetime of these bad health habits? Why do intelligent people willingly immerse themselves in these lethal practices?

Part of the answer involves self-responsibility. Traditionally we have been conditioned to think that someone else is responsible for our health or state of wellness. We never stop to consider the end result of a life of bad health habits. We just keep on indulging. But only one person is responsible for your wellness—and that is you. It is your responsibility to carefully evaluate each of your negative lifestyles so that you can be aware of the disastrous end results. This book provides detailed information and a Personal Plan which will allow you to understand and comprehend your own wellness responsibility and enable you to accept it and take control of your own well-being.

The second reason millions of people continue with a life full of negative lifestyles is simple: changing bad health habits is not easy! As a matter of fact, in most cases, people have tried to eliminate their bad health habits and *failed.* By studying not failure but *success,* we have been able to develop and perfect the "Plan for the Elimination of Negative Lifestyles." This Plan will work for you. The Plan is described and personalized for you in this book. If you read this book and study and apply the Plan correctly and diligently, you will achieve the ultimate results—you *will* feel better and you *will* live longer.

The single most important working factor in achieving high-level wellness is the thought process. The reason most people fail to eliminate their negative lifestyles is because they neglect to harness their thought processes. They fail to call forth their most potent ally—Mind Power. This book shows you *how* to use your Mind Power in the revolutionary technique of *visualization*. By using the simple technique of visualization, you will be able to conquer any of the harmful health habits you choose.

This book is divided into two parts. Book One provides you with general information on the subject of wellness and explains in detail how the process of visualization is used in the Plan for the Elimination of Negative Lifestyles.

The second part, Book Two, is actually six books in one. A separate chapter is devoted to overcoming each of the six most harmful health habits. They are smoking, the inability to cope with everyday stress, poor nutrition, obesity, excessive consumption of alcohol, and the lack of physical fitness. Each chapter is a complete, self-contained program. Everything required for you to eliminate your bad health habits forever is included.

You are about to become involved in the most important activity of your lifetime. You are going to take charge of your own health destiny. You are going to assure yourself of maximum longevity and enhanced quality of life. You will soon erase from your life one of the greatest hazards of this generation—*premature death.*

I wish you every success on your journey to the ultimate in life: WELLNESS—FEELING BETTER AND LIVING LONGER.

R. WILLIAM WHITMER
EXECUTIVE DIRECTOR
WELLNESS CENTERS OF AMERICA, INC.
P.O. BOX 76082
BIRMINGHAM, ALABAMA 35223

BOOK ONE

1. THE WELLNESS RENAISSANCE

"All glory comes from daring to begin."
E. F. WARE

At one time I weighed 205 pounds. I now weigh 159, which is ideal for my height, age, and body configuration. A number of years ago I could not run around a city block without stopping to rest. Now I compete in numerous 10,000-meter races. Once I was hospitalized for extensive tests after it was discovered that my blood pressure was dangerously high. My blood pressure now averages 130/82. In the not too distant past, I rarely went through a day without consuming a considerable amount of alcohol. Now it's an occasional beer or glass of wine. Previously, I had a real problem with everyday stress. Always on the run, really thinking the world would crumble if I stopped. I now have an entirely different outlook on life. A while back my eating habits were a dietician's nightmare. Too much fat, cholesterol, sugar, salt, and too many calories. Now, I'm monitoring my diet carefully and am very content. Two packs of cigarettes used to be my daily minimum. Now, I don't smoke.

Sound unreasonable or impossible? Yes, but it shouldn't. Few people are aware that such dramatic changes can be made in their lives. In a country with a population as sophisticated and intelligent as ours, only five of each one hundred people have an in-depth working knowledge of *how* and *why* behavior and lifestyles affect one's health. However, this is about to change.

A new era of interest in improved personal health is sweeping across the nation. At no time in history have so many expressed such a sincere desire to become actively involved in programs which allow them to take charge of their own health. Today people are no longer content to sit back and let diseases and illnesses occur at random. Now they want to be a part of their own health destiny.

What has caused this upsurge in personal interest to stay well? There are two main reasons. First, what's happening is a natural extension of the "exercise craze" which started in the 1970s. At that time tens of millions of people started and have remained on programs for physical fitness. Now, many have reached peak physical condition and have started asking: Where do I go from here? The satisfaction derived from top physical conditioning has caused curiosity about self-improvement in other areas of health. Those who have had a taste of good health want more.

The second reason for the escalating interest in staying well is because the population is becoming better informed about medical and health matters. We are constantly exposed to health-related information through books, television, radio, and newspapers. Numerous prestigious organizations such as the American Heart Association, the American Cancer Society, and the President's Council on Fitness and Sports Medicine conduct highly successful public information campaigns to increase awareness. These and other groups have pointed out the following:

> If people didn't smoke, at least 80 percent of the 98,000 annual deaths from lung cancer, cancer of the larynx, mouth, and esophagus would be prevented. Lung cancer is not the only disease linked to smoking. According to a recent study, the mortality from heart disease is 3.6 times higher in smokers as compared to nonsmokers.
>
> If people cut down on the consumption of animal fat, exercised more, and didn't smoke, the annual death rate from heart attacks—638,000—would be considerably decreased.
>
> If people curbed their salt intake and didn't smoke, the yearly deaths due to strokes—183,000—would be cut significantly.
>
> Cutting down on the amount of food consumed is another way to cut down on premature deaths. If all the obesity in the population was eliminated, it would probably have the greatest impact on increasing life-span.
>
> Improper diet is a prime factor in promoting serious illness and premature deaths. Yearly consumption of sugar in this country is 120 lbs. per capita. This carbohydrate intake contributes to obesity and hypoglycemia and increases blood clotting tendencies which can lead to coronary thrombosis.
>
> Regular exercise primes the immune system (the cells and antibodies that protect us against disease) and helps our brain and body resist aging. If human brain and body are kept in good condition, they deteriorate less rapidly.

Statements like these have caused many people to want to know more. As they learn more, they start asking questions.

I travel extensively, conducting Wellness Seminars for large corporations and for communities through hospital sponsorship. Almost on a daily basis, I come in contact with hundreds of people who are interested in health self-improvement. Based upon this experience, I am aware of the questions being asked.

Smokers know there is a warning statement on every pack of cigarettes, but what does this mean to the individual? Is he or she really going to get lung cancer? What about emphysema or other acute or chronic lung diseases? Most people know that excessive alcohol is harmful, but how about in moderation? How much is too much? Many realize that a regular exercise program is good, but how much exercise and how often? And what can be done about the stress that surrounds us most of the time? How harmful is it to be overweight? How can a person start on a diet and stay with it? Should attempts be made to limit cholesterol? How about HDL and LDL? Will fiber prevent certain kinds of cancer?

These and dozens of other questions are the result of unprecedented interest in personal health. This high-level interest is the beginning of a new era which is becoming known as the *Wellness Renaissance*. The Wellness Renaissance is based upon the discovery that the human body is one of the most responsive organisms on earth. It responds in direct proportion to how it is treated. The body which is abused, misused, and neglected malfunctions more often and wears out faster. This means the body ages quicker and dies sooner. On the other hand, the body which is cared for and taken care of has less problems. It suffers less breakdowns and lasts longer. The aging process slows down and life-span increases. It's that simple.

NEGATIVE LIFESTYLES AND RISK FACTORS

Daily activities that reflect how you care for or neglect your body are called lifestyles or risk factors. Let's consider a few of them here.

A risk factor is any condition, situation, or activity which increases the possibility of the development of a clinical disease. Risk factors may be divided into three types: the uncontrollable, the semicontrollable, and the controllable.

An example of an uncontrollable risk factor would be heredity. Our genes may predispose us toward certain diseases. The hereditary diseases we hear about most often are diabetes and cardiovascular diseases. Heredity is a risk factor over which we have no control. We cannot choose our parents and, therefore, if one or both parents had a specific hereditary disease, we must accept the higher risk of developing this same disease. This is not to suggest that genetically communicated diseases will always occur. The individual who is interested in wellness and knows he or she is predisposed to a disease will try to do something about it. For example, the "wellness"-oriented person whose mother and/or father have diabetes will not just lie back with the attitude that diabetes is inevitable. This person learns everything possible about diabetes, avoids becoming overweight, and restricts carbohydrate intake, because this may delay the onset of the disease.

Other uncontrollable risk factors are age and sex. The older you become, the more likely you are to develop certain diseases. With regard to sex, males are usually more predisposed to develop some diseases than females. This is true in conditions such as hypertension and heart attacks.

The semicontrollable risk factor can be illustrated by environmental conditions. Often the workplace or the air in general may be polluted to the point of being a risk factor. Though improvements have been made, this is still a major problem in some areas. We refer to this as a semicontrollable risk factor because it is one that *can* be eliminated even though often it's not practical to do so.

The vast majority of health risk factors are completely controllable. Experts have estimated that 85 percent of our risk factors are controllable. Some of the more common controllable risk factors are:

- smoking
- obesity
- poor nutrition
- stress
- lack of regular exercise
- excessive consumption of alcohol

Throughout this book, I refer to negative lifestyles. It is important for you to understand that the terms *risk factor* and *negative lifestyle* can usually be used interchangeably. A negative lifestyle is always a risk factor. However, risk factors such as heredity, age, and sex are not negative lifestyles.

PREMATURE DEATH

Any consideration of risk factors or negative lifestyles can be a difficult subject because they are by nature somewhat nebulous. Do negative lifestyles really have an effect on one's life? One way to answer this is to look at one of the most topical subjects in today's medical literature: *premature death.*

The study of risk factors or negative lifestyles is of extreme interest to insurance companies as they update and prepare actuary tables. These companies have studied tens of thousands of people with a variety of negative lifestyles and are now able to accurately predict the number of years of life you will lose due to each negative lifestyle.

I would like to share with you the latest information available from insurance companies and other sources about premature death. This information is taken directly from their actuary tables. (It is important to understand that any time you use actuary tables, you are using averages. There are always exceptions to every average.)

- For every ten pounds you are overweight, you will die two years sooner when compared to a person of ideal body weight.
- Consider two men aged fifty. One has never smoked. The other has smoked one or more packs of cigarettes a day for the past thirty years. The smoker, according to averages, will die eight and a half years sooner than the nonsmoker.
- How about hypertension, the silent killer? There are two men aged fifty-five. One has a blood pressure of 120/80, which is considered normal. The other has a blood pressure of 180/100, which is high blood pressure. If the individual with high blood pressure does not bring it under control, he will die eleven and a half years earlier than the person with controlled or normal blood pressure.
- Consider elevated cholesterol in the blood. One person has a blood cholesterol of less than 194 mg. %. The other has a blood cholesterol of 250 mg. % or more. The individual with the higher blood cholesterol level has a three times greater chance of developing cardiovascular diseases, primarily a stroke or heart attack.
- Consider excessive daily consumption of large amounts of alcohol. It has been estimated that the chronic (daily) heavy drinker will die eight years sooner than the nondrinker or light drinker.

Data such as these are available on numerous risk factors and negative lifestyles. They always come to the same conclusion: certain negative lifestyles subtract years from your life-span.

Usually when individuals hear about premature death for the first time, they become concerned or frightened or skeptical. Those who are skeptical may tell the story of a person they knew personally who smoked three packs of cigarettes a day, drank a quart of whiskey, had high blood pressure, and lived to be eighty-nine years old. We all know of a person who fits this pattern. This proves that the actuary tables from which we obtain data on premature death are based on averages, and the old-timer mentioned above is the exception. But more to the point, we all also know of the too familiar cases in which a forty-two-year-old man with hypertension died or is paralyzed from a stroke, or the forty-five-year-old smoker who died of lung cancer, or the fifty-year-old person who has not been involved in regular exercise since college and has had triple bypass coronary surgery.

Premature death is real. It is a recognized clinical entity. As the Wellness Renaissance develops, increasing numbers of people are becoming informed and educated about premature death. Having knowledge about premature death, knowing what causes it and, most importantly, how to prevent it, is what the Wellness Renaissance is all about.

CARDIOVASCULAR DISEASE RISK FACTORS

We probably know more about the relationship between risk factors and cardiovascular diseases than any other medical condition. According to the American Heart Association, in 1978 nearly one million people died from cardiovascular diseases. Fifty-two percent of all deaths in the United States were caused by this problem.

I would like to present these data to you in a different way. During a given year, more people die of cardiovascular (CV) diseases than all other causes combined, including murders, suicides, and accidents. Frightening, isn't it? It should be. But it is also vitally important for you to understand that you have direct control over all the risk factors which predispose you to CV diseases, except heredity, age, and sex.

The controllable ones are smoking, obesity, lack of regular exercise, poor nutrition, and stress. These are exactly the same risk factors or negative lifestyles that I can help you eliminate. If you are successful in eliminating these negative lifestyles, the chances of preventing CV diseases, increasing your life-span, and enhancing the quality of your life will become a reality for you.

The concern about CV diseases is such that numerous, simple risk factor (negative lifestyle) charts have been formulated which allow you to predict the possibility of developing CV diseases.

One of the best I have seen was developed by the Michigan Heart Association. It is presented in the form of a game called Risko.

RISKO

The purpose of this game is to give you an estimate of your chances of suffering heart attack.

The game is played by making squares which—from left to right—represent an increase in your risk factors. These are medical conditions and habits associated with an increased danger of heart attack. Not all risk factors are measurable enough to be included in Risko. (See page 10.)

Rules:
Study each risk factor and its row. Find the box applicable to you and circle the large number in it. For example, if you are thirty-seven, circle the number in the box labeled 31–40. After checking out all the rows, add the circled numbers. The total—your score—is an estimate of your risk.

Heredity:
Count parents, grandparents, brothers, and sisters who have had a heart attack and/or a stroke.

Tobacco smoking:
If you inhale deeply and smoke a cigarette way down, add one to your classification. Do NOT subtract because you think you do not inhale or smoke only a half inch of a cigarette.

Exercise:
Lower your score one point if you exercise regularly and frequently.

Cholesterol or saturated fat intake level:
A cholesterol blood level check is best. If you can't get one from your physician, then estimate honestly the percentage of solid fats you eat. These are usually of animal origin—eggs, lard, cream, butter, beef, and lamb. If you eat much of this, your cholesterol level may be high.

Blood pressure:
If you have no recent reading but have passed an insurance or industrial examination, chances are you are 140 or less.

Sex:
This line takes into account the fact that men have from six to ten times more heart attacks than women of child-bearing age.

RISKO

AGE	10 to 20 **1**	21 to 30 **2**	31 to 40 **3**	41 to 50 **4**	51 to 60 **6**	61 to 70 and over **8**
HEREDITY	No known history of heart disease **1**	1 relative with cardiovascular disease Over 60 **2**	2 relatives with cardiovascular disease Over 60 **3**	1 relative with cardiovascular disease Under 60 **4**	2 relatives with cardiovascular disease Under 60 **6**	3 relatives with cardiovascular disease Under 60 **7**
WEIGHT	More than 5 lbs. below standard weight **0**	−5 to +5 lbs. standard weight **1**	6-20 lbs. over weight **2**	21-35 lbs. over weight **3**	36-50 lbs. over weight **5**	51-65 lbs. over weight **7**
TOBACCO SMOKING	non-user **0**	Cigar and/or pipe **1**	10 cigarettes or less a day **2**	20 cigarettes a day **4**	30 cigarettes a day **6**	40 cigarettes a day or more **10**
EXERCISE	Intensive occupational and recreational exertion **1**	Moderate occupational and recreational exertion **2**	Sedentary work and intense recreational exertion **3**	Sedentary occupational and moderate recreational exertion **5**	Sedentary work and light recreational exertion **6**	Complete lack of all exercise **8**
CHOLESTEROL OR FAT % IN DIET	below 180 mg. Diet contains no animal or solid fats **1**	Cholestrerol 181-205 mg. Diet contains 10% animal or solid fats **2**	Cholesterol 206-230 mg. Diet contains 20% animal or solid fats **3**	Cholesterol 231-255 mg. Diet contains 30% animal or solid fats **4**	Cholesterol 256-280 mg. Diet contains 40% animal or solid fats **5**	Cholesterol 281-300 mg. Diet contains 50% animal or solid fats **7**
BLOOD PRESSURE	100 upper reading **1**	120 upper reading **2**	140 upper reading **3**	160 upper reading **4**	180 upper reading **6**	200 or over upper reading **8**
SEX	Female under 40 **1**	Female 40-50 **2**	Female over 50 **3**	Male **5**	Stocky male **6**	Bald stocky male **7**

If you score:

6–11	Risk well below average	25–31	Risk moderately high
12–17	Risk below average	31–40	Risk at a dangerous level
18–24	Risk generally average	41–62	Danger urgent. See your physician now!

Because of the difficulty in measuring them, the following risk factors are not included in Risko:

- Diabetes, particularly when present for many years.
- Your character or personality, and the stress under which you live.
- Your vital capacity, which is determined by measuring the amount of air you can take into your lungs in proportion to the size of your lungs. The less air you can breathe, the higher your risk.
- Abnormalities in an electrocardiogram. If certain abnormalities are present in the record of the electrical currents generated by your heart you have a higher risk.
- Gout, which is caused by a higher-than-normal amount of uric acid in the blood. Patients have an increased risk.

The Michigan Heart Association recommends: "If you have a number of risk factors, for the sake of your health, ask your doctor to check your medical condition, and quit your risk factor habits. Note: The fact that various habits or conditions may be rated similarly in this test does not mean these are of equal risk. The reaction of individual human beings to risk factors—as to many other things—is so varied it is impossible to draw valid conclusions for any individual. This scale has been developed only to highlight what the risk factors are and what can be done about them. It is not designed to be a medical diagnosis."

THE DEVELOPMENT OF WELLNESS

Do you take illness for granted? Most people do. Many have the attitude that illness is a part of living and each of us is allocated a certain amount. It's our lot in life and little can be done to alter or change the amount or degree of illness that affects each of us.

Do you fit into this pattern? Perhaps you have never given thought to the actual control you have over encouraging or preventing illness within your own life.

In the United States, as in all Western countries and Japan, the health care delivery system is directed primarily toward the treatment and cure of illness. The medical education system, the fee for service system, the mechanism for paying for health services, and the structure of the hospital system itself are all oriented toward treatment and cure.

This is great, but what about preventing disease?

With the sophisticated advances in today's medical know-how, it is often overlooked that the single most dramatic advance in medicine has been prevention. Immunization and sanitation, which protect us from contracting a disease, have become, during this century, widespread forms of preventive medicine. Prevention has played a major role in reducing illness and deaths due to contagious diseases.

Preventive medicine is a concept whose time has come not only for contagious diseases, but also for chronic diseases. The best way to combat such diseases is to prevent their occurring in the first place.

What is preventive medicine? Preventive medicine includes programs that attempt to eliminate a disease completely. It also includes the attempt to detect a disease before it is symptomatic. (The Pap smear is an example.) Preventive medicine includes those efforts to control and/or reduce the effects of a condition. (Examples are diabetes control and the management of hypertension.)

What is the relationship between preventive medicine and wellness? Preventive medicine is a part of wellness. As you become involved in high-level wellness, you must be aware of the proven and traditional methods of preventive medicine and incorporate them into your program.

Several years ago, I attended a Preventive Medicine Conference. The following story was told by a physician who was a Preventive Medicine specialist:

> A medical convention was taking place in a city which was located on a large river. The Convention Center was adjacent to the river. During a break in the meeting, a young physician took a walk along the river. He had not gone more than five minutes when he heard the cries of a person who was obviously drowning. Being an excellent swimmer, the physician jumped into the river, swam to the person in distress and pulled him ashore. On the river bank the physician expertly resuscitated the patient. No sooner was this person resuscitated than the physician heard a second cry for help. Without a moment's delay, he again jumped into the river and pulled a second person out. After reviving this person, yet a third was heard calling for help. Although somewhat exhausted, the physician again went into the water and, with some difficulty, made it to the river bank. After the third near-drowning victim was saved, a second young physician came on the scene and, upon learning what had happened, heard a fourth per-

son cry for help. Aware of what had taken place, the second physician asked the first, "Why don't we find out why so many people are falling in the river so we can stop it?" As the first physician again started for the river, he yelled over his shoulder, "No, let's save them all!"

Unfortunately, this simple story illustrates the attitude of many in the health care profession toward preventive medicine, health promotion, health enhancement, and wellness: "Call me when there is a problem and I will come immediately. However, prevention is not what I devote my energies and talents to."

THE ILLNESS CONTINUUM

Traditionally we have always thought of illness and wellness as opposites. This is not true. The two are related. As a matter of fact, illness and wellness are one continuum.

Let's look at the illness part of the continuum first, as illustrated below.

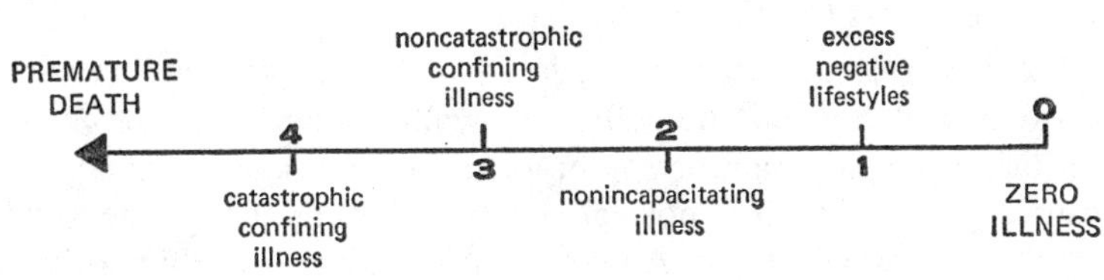

THE ILLNESS CONTINUUM

The right end of the line is *zero,* which means the person is without illness or, by traditional thinking, well.

Level 1 on the Illness Continuum is reached when you engage regularly in negative lifestyles. You may be asymptomatic most of the time, but you are definitely heading in the wrong direction. The illustration on page 14 depicts two of my friends at this level. They are practicing the Five Deadly S's—smoking, sitting, snacks, sugar, and salt.

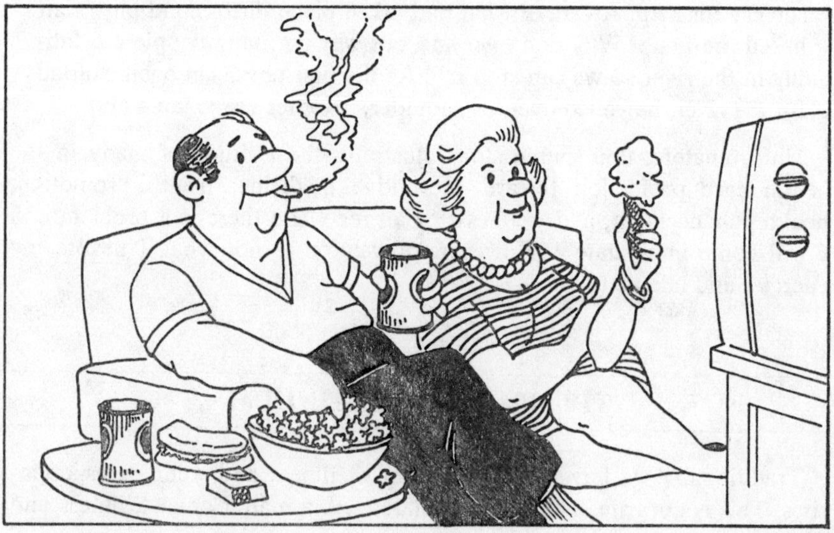

The Five Deadly S's

In addition, they are overweight and he may consume too much alcohol. Few people, using traditional definitions, would consider my friends ill, but on the Illness Continuum they are.

Level 2 on the Illness Continuum is a stopping place, on occasion, for many people and is when you suffer any acute illness. It could be a case of sinusitus, a muscle strain or spasm, or a common cold. It is any illness that causes you not to feel normal but not sick enough to be confined throughout the day and night. Anyone can find himself at this position on the Illness Continuum. The main difference between a person with high-level wellness and one without is the speed with which he returns to zero on the continuum. Returning to zero is greatly affected by the number of negative lifestyles (level 1). Put another way, a high-level wellness person recovers and recuperates faster and more thoroughly.

Level 3 is reached when you are confined at home or at the hospital with a self-limiting medical condition. This might be for surgery for appendicitis, in traction for a broken bone, or at home with pneumonia. Usually, immediately following the confinement, you will pass through level 2. Again, the time spent at level 2 on the return to zero will depend on the number and severity of the excessive negative lifestyles in which you indulge (level 1).

Level 4 is reached when there is a truly life-threatening condition, such as lung cancer or heart attack. It is a proven fact that level 1 can play an important part in getting to level 4. For example, there is a clear cause-effect relationship between chronic, heavy smoking and lung diseases. According to our continuum, during the life of a heavy smoker there may be acute, then chronic coughing (level 2). Emphysema may develop along with acute or chronic pulmonary infections (levels 2 and 3). Finally, cancer is diagnosed (level 4). The smoker who is interested in high-level wellness must understand that cancer does not occur overnight. There are predictable and reproduceable events on the Illness Continuum that may eventually end up as cancer.

All risk factors (negative lifestyles) that predispose a person to a heart attack—our leading cause of death—start at level 1, except for heredity, age, and sex. These predisposing factors are smoking, obesity, stress, poor nutrition, and lack of regular exercise. These can cause a variety of diseases of the circulatory system such as angina and atherosclerosis. Angina can be acute or chronic; it can be transient or incapacitating (levels 2 and 3). The only thing for sure is that it can be the forerunner of a heart attack and premature death.

The main point is that illness is usually not a singular symptomatic event. It is a predictable, moving phenomenon which ranges from a zero point through a number of levels to premature death. In order to achieve high-level wellness, it is essential that you have a thorough understanding of the Illness Continuum.

WHAT IS WELLNESS?

For most people, it is more difficult to define wellness than illness. All of us at one time or another have been ill. We know what happens and how we feel. Wellness is something else. Many people I have talked with think that if you are not ill, then you are well. For many, the most frequent definition of being well is not being sick. So, where does wellness fit into the picture?

To begin with, wellness is the realization and acceptance of wellness self-responsibility. Next, wellness is the reduction and then elimination of all your negative health habits. This means stop smoking, consume moderate amounts of alcohol or none at all, arrive at and maintain ideal body weight, exercise regularly, consume a well-balanced diet, and learn to cope with everyday stress.

Another dimension of wellness lies in introspection, or getting to know one's self. This emotional or spiritual part of wellness develops when wellness responsibility is accepted and negative lifestyles are eliminated. As attention is diverted from blatant pleasure-producing activities such as smoking, eating, imbibing, and the sedentary life, it is easier to concentrate on one's internal life.

At this point, I would like to share with you the very simple definition of wellness that I have developed. You will find my definition shorter and less complicated than most. If you accept it, assimilate it, make it a part of you, then you can grow to the acceptance of other, more lengthy and complex definitions.

- Wellness is taking aggressive, positive action rather than a passive role in dictating and directing your health destiny.
- Wellness is total comprehension and acceptance of your own responsibility for staying well.
- Wellness is the systematic recognition and elimination of all your negative lifestyles.
- Wellness is a way of life which results in maximum longevity and enhanced quality of life.
- Wellness is feeling better and living longer.

As you develop and mature in your wellness growth cycle, you may want to add to this definition. That's great. The more you become involved, the more successful you will be.

THE WELLNESS CONTINUUM

Just as there is an Illness Continuum, there is also a Wellness Continuum. Like the Illness Continuum, the Wellness Continuum is not static but dynamic and ever-moving.

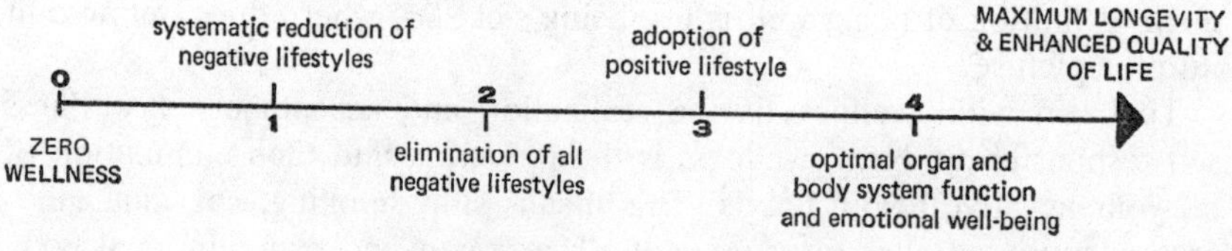

THE WELLNESS CONTINUUM

On the left side of the continuum is *zero* wellness, which is basically an asymptomatic but far from high-level wellness situation.

To the right of zero is **level 1,** which is the recognition and systematic reduction of your negative lifestyles. It is important to have a level for this activity because most people have multinegative lifestyles (more than one). The greatest mistake is for you to become so enthusiastic about wellness that you attempt to eliminate all your negative lifestyles at one time. They must be eliminated one at a time, as will be explained in Book Two.

Level 2 is reached when you have successfully eliminated all your harmful health practices. You can make some allowances for situations in which it is impossible to completely eliminate the harmful activity. For example, a person who travels extensively may have some difficulty in constantly remaining on the ideal balanced diet. However, this should not detract from *trying* to completely eliminate all negative lifestyles.

Level 3 is reached when you reorganize your life to implement a positive lifestyle. By the very nature of eliminating lifestyles such as smoking, consuming excessive alcohol, indifference to regular exercise, obesity, poor nutrition, and the inability to cope with stress, you start to adopt a positive lifestyle. Included in level 3 is introspection—getting to know one's self from the inside out, so that your new wellness attitude can become a reality. Level 3 involves the emotional or spiritual aspects of wellness.

Level 4 becomes a reality only after considerable time and effort. It takes practice and patience. It means *treating your life as if it is truly your most prized and valued possession.* It is achieved only after elimination or concentrated reduction of all your negative lifestyles, as well as realization of your new self-awareness. After achieving level 4, a person is assured of maximum life-span and enhanced quality of life. Stated another way, it is the assurance of feeling better and living longer.

THE ILLNESS-WELLNESS CONTINUUM

The Illness Continuum and the Wellness Continuum are not separate but join to create the Illness-Wellness Continuum, as below:

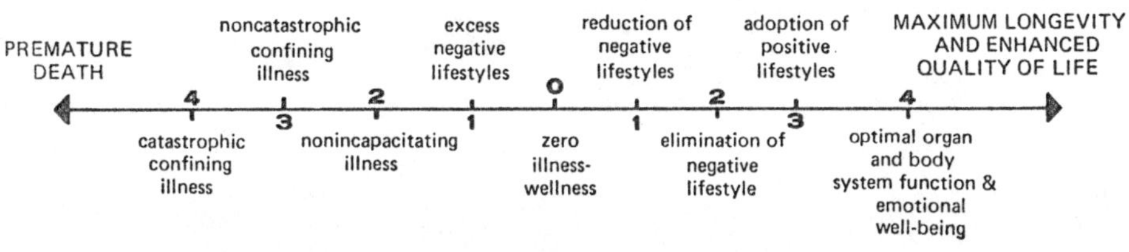

THE ILLNESS - WELLNESS CONTINUUM

Due to external and internal factors, you may find yourself moving back and forth on the continuum. It is possible for you to be on the far right of the wellness side of the continuum and still become ill and move to the left, on the illness side. However, the further you are to the right in the beginning, the faster will be your return to the right.

As can be seen from the Illness-Wellness Continuum, illness is not an all-or-nothing situation. There are degrees of illness leading to premature death. The progression down the Illness Continuum, in many instances, is controllable. Wellness is strongly influenced by external factors, which you can control to maximize your life-span and enhance the quality of your life.

The discovery and understanding of the Illness-Wellness Continuum can be one of the most significant discoveries of a lifetime. By understanding this concept, you can add pleasurable *extra* years of good health to your life. You can control your own health destiny by personally manipulating your own position on the Illness-Wellness Continuum. Adding years to your life and enhancing the quality of your life are strictly up to you. If you are interested, then take your next step toward your own WELLNESS RENAISSANCE.

2. WELLNESS IS YOUR RESPONSIBILITY —DON'T DENY IT!

"The vast majority of persons
have a natural tendency
to shrink from the responsibility
of standing and acting alone."
FRANCIS GALTON

When considering the recipe for high-level wellness, self-responsibility accounts for 50 percent of the ingredients.

Few are aware of this fact because traditionally we have been conditioned to assume that the responsibility for our staying well belongs to someone else. We now know that this is not true. Your physician can advise you to stop smoking and inform you of the possible consequences if you don't, but he or she cannot make you stop smoking. Only *you* can do that. If you have high blood pressure, your physician can prescribe medicine and a diet, your husband or wife or someone else can constantly remind you to take the pills and avoid salt, but *you* make the decision about taking the medicine and staying on the diet. You can buy and read one of the many books on exercise programs but only *you* can decide to follow it. You can become an expert on the various methods of meditation to control stress but only *you* can arrange your schedule to devote the required time to your form of relaxation. You can have a dozen people—from your physician to your best friend—tell you that you should lose weight but only *you* can start on the proper diet and stay on it. Even though you are well aware of the hazards of excessive alcohol, only *you* can make the decision to eliminate or reduce alcohol as a part of your everyday life. The responsibility for your wellness belongs to *you—no one else—you!*

We know the basic problem in getting people to realize their own responsibility for high-level wellness. The following will illustrate.

Not long ago, I was in a large bookstore in one of our major cities. In the course of browsing, I came across a list of the ten best-selling books in the country. Three of the ten best-sellers were on the general subject of health. Two concerned themselves with diet and the third was about physical fitness. When you stop to think about it, this is incredible. Thirty-three percent of the best-selling nonfiction books in the country are on the subject of health, that is, eliminating negative lifestyles.

One conclusion can be drawn from so much reading about lifestyle change, wellness concepts, and all the other activities we know are happening (jogging, obesity clinics, the boon in health spa registration, and more): *people want to assume greater responsibility for their own health and wellness, but the problem is, they don't know how.* Learning the importance of responsibility and how to assume it is a major part of the Wellness Renaissance.

When considering self-responsibility, it is important to understand that wellness self-responsibility does not mean antiphysician. I stress this because some so-called wellness programs emphasize self-diagnosis and self-treatment. They deemphasize or demean the role of the physician and the professional health care team. They are of the opinion that we are over-diagnosed, overtested, and overtreated. They point out that the majority of diseases are self-limiting and that the body has a magnificent ability to cure itself of many illnesses. No one can deny there is some truth in these statements, but to ignore the physician is a recipe for certain disaster.

The physician is needed for regular physical examinations as well as for when you are truly ill. With this observation, the question is: Can the physician play a major role in helping you to achieve high-level wellness? The answer is usually *no.* Because of the busy schedule of most physicians, they do not have time to become involved with in-depth patient education and motivation. Without information and motivation, you will not be able to accept full responsibility. Without acceptance of your own health responsibilities, you will not be able to eliminate your bad health habits. Unless negative lifestyles are eliminated, there is no possibility for you to achieve high-level wellness.

I have discussed wellness and health responsibility with thousands of people across the United States. Invariably there is a paradox. I have found that people who have high levels of responsibility in nearly all facets of their lives will almost never have any for their own health and wellness. Are you in this group? If so, you stand with the overwhelming majority.

Why do most people ignore this, perhaps the most important of all responsibilities? The reasons are:

1) *Lack of information and knowledge.* Most people do not have the basic training or understanding of health, illness, and wellness to realize their responsibility. You cannot respond to any situation

in a responsible manner without understandable facts. Basic information about body function, illness, disease, treatment, and prognosis have not been readily available until recent years.

People are realizing that with more information they can assume greater responsibility. However, it is important to point out that there is a big difference between information and knowledge.

Having information is simply being aware of the fact that certain data exist. For example, when a smoker reads the statement on a pack of cigarettes—"smoking is dangerous to your health"—that's information. Information becomes knowledge when it is fully comprehended and when it becomes meaningful to the individual. When the smoker truly comprehends *how* and *why* it is harmful to *him* or *her,* and the calculated *personal* health risk it presents, the information becomes knowledge.

Experience has proved beyond a doubt that there is a definite ratio between increased knowledge and the willingness and desire to assume greater responsibility for personal wellness.

2) *Lack of belief or realization.* Many people still do not believe that catastrophic illness, premature aging, premature death, or other serious problems can occur to *them* because of negative lifestyles.

The smoker always thinks: "I can never get lung cancer. It may happen to my friends but never to me." The individual with high blood pressure who does not take prescribed medication or stay on the diet provided by the physician is sure he will never have a stroke. "It may happen to my friends but never to me." The obese person who has not exercised regularly in years is positive he will not have a heart attack. "It may happen to my friends but never to me."

Though it sounds like a broken record, the fact is: if a person really knew about the direct correlation and proved connection between negative lifestyles and premature death and understood that no one is exempt, negative lifestyles would never be practiced again.

3) *Lack of motivation.* People must be motivated in order to change behavioral patterns and lifestyles. The problem is that our present health care system devotes virtually no time or money to educating or motivating people. There is even less energy and resources expended to inform and teach people *how* to eliminate negative lifestyles. People must be motivated in order to assume wellness self-responsibility.

A word about motivation is in order. Motivation is an

internal phenomenon. It must come from within. I cannot motivate you, nor can anyone else. What I can do is *stimulate* you to motivate yourself. Once you are really stimulated, you will motivate yourself as never before. You will become enthusiastic about your own wellness as you become convinced that you have the power to increase your life-span and to enhance the quality of your life.

This book is your answer to learning *how* to accept your responsibility for your wellness. It contains a tremendous amount of information with instructions on *how* to convert it into personal knowledge. Data is presented which will convince you to believe and realize that premature aging and death are real and that negative lifestyles can cause them to detract from your life-span and the quality of life. This book is a powerful influence for stimulating you to motivate yourself toward high-level wellness.

Once people are informed and stimulated, things start to happen. They become motivated to want to stop smoking, lose weight, be more relaxed, consume less alcohol, eat a more nutritious diet, and get more exercise. The reason for this is probably subconscious. Once the mind understands and comprehends responsibility, it reacts accordingly. This is one of the most potent factors behind the motivation to start down and stay on the road to high-level wellness.

Now you are ready to learn the revolutionary technique of VISUALIZATION to help you motivate yourself and to help inform you in a way you will find impossible to forget. Then you will move to the chapters that will show you new and foolproof techniques which will enable you to conquer your bad health habits. All this is possible now that you know and understand that WELLNESS IS YOUR RESPONSIBILITY. DON'T DENY IT!

3. USING VISUALIZATION AND THE THOUGHT PROCESS TO FEEL BETTER AND LIVE LONGER

"Bring ideas in and entertain them royally, for one of them may be king."
MARK VAN DOREN

The human brain is the most complex piece of matter in the universe. A computer sophisticated enough to process the functions of a single brain cell would more than cover the face of the earth. The brain is made up of over ten billion such cells.

The mind, which is the function of the brain, exists at two distinct levels—the conscious and the subconscious.

The conscious mind functions when you are awake and aware of sensations, thoughts, the environment, and your own existence. When you are asleep or for some other reason unconscious, the conscious mind ceases to function. The other part of your mind, the subconscious, is different in that it functions all the time, twenty-four hours a day, whether you are asleep or awake.

Because the conscious mind is dominant, many people are not aware of what the subconscious mind is, what it does, and what it can do. Even though you may be in this group you have probably experienced the functioning of your own subconscious mind in numerous ways. For example, have you ever been in the situation of having to get up in the morning at a time different from your normal routine? Let's say your usual time for rising is 6 A.M., but because of something special, you must get up at 5:15. What happens in many cases? At precisely 5:15, without the alarm clock, you suddenly wake up. What causes this to happen? Through your planning and anticipation you have consciously or unconsciously instructed your subconscious mind to wake the conscious mind at 5:15.

Many mothers have had the experience of being instantly waked from a deep sleep by the slightest sound made by the baby in another room.

Why is this? After all, the baby is some distance away and the noise is so slight that it should not even be heard much less wake a person who is sleeping. The subconscious mind never sleeps. In this case, because of the mother's concern for the baby, the subconscious mind is listening. When the baby whimpers, the subconscious mind wakes the conscious mind and the mother is instantly aware of the noise.

The subconscious mind controls many of the functions of your body. Through the autonomic nervous system, important factors such as heart rate, respiration, secretion of digestive enzymes, blood pressure, and many other activities are regulated with no input from the conscious mind. When you go to sleep, you don't have to think about or provide any conscious instructions to ensure that your heart will beat a certain number of times per minute. It isn't necessary to issue thought instructions for your lungs to breathe on a regular basis. If you ate an orange before going to bed, you don't need to be consciously concerned about the complex digestive process which works while you are asleep. All these functions and many more are controlled by the subconscious mind.

Since the subconscious mind plays such an important role in your life, the big question is: *How can you influence your subconscious mind?*

There are two ways. One is by your thoughts. What you think has tremendous influence over your subconscious. However, the most effective way is by *visualization.*

So much is being said and written about visualization. What is it?

Visualization is the creation of, then concentration on a specific and detailed mental picture.

For reasons which will be explained later, high-level wellness *must* begin in the subconscious mind. Visualization is the bridge which spans the gap between your conscious and subconscious mind. It is the method by which you communicate with your subconscious mind as often as you want.

Now that you know what visualization is, I would like to reflect back and share with you how the discovery was made of the influence the thought process and visualization can have over the subconscious and why they are absolutely essential for high-level wellness.

WHY YOU FAIL

When I started to develop a Plan which would assure high-level wellness, one of the first questions asked was: Is there a common factor, a universal thread which weaves itself throughout the lives of those with negative lifestyles? After extensive study, I can tell you: Yes, there is a common or universal factor.

The one thing that people with negative behavioral patterns all have in common is simply *failure*. Individuals with negative lifestyles have often tried to eliminate them on their own and they have failed. Let's look at a few facts. Seventy-nine percent of the people in the United States who smoke have conscientiously tried on at least one occasion to stop and they have failed. Seventy-one percent of the people who are overweight have gone on a diet at least once, lost a significant amount of weight, and gained it back. They have failed. Sixty-eight percent of the people who are enthusiastic and start out on a program of regular exercise are no longer exercising within thirty days. They have failed.

I could go on with other examples. Suffice it to say, most individuals who have negative lifestyles have tried to eliminate them but for a variety of reasons have failed.

Once it was discovered that failure is common to a life filled with negative lifestyles, the question was raised: Can the secret to conquering negative lifestyles be found in a study of that activity which is the exact opposite of failure—*success?*

Can the reason for success be defined? Is there a dependable, reproduceable formula which can be used to turn failure into success? I am pleased to tell you that the answer is yes. There are time-tested methods for achieving success and *they have been transposed into a Plan for the Elimination of Negative Lifestyles.* This information can be the most important discovery of your life. Can you think of anything more important than feeling better and living longer?

When I started my journey to find the formula for success in achieving high-level wellness, I was attracted to work done by the late Napoleon Hill. When Napoleon Hill was a young man, he was introduced to Andrew Carnegie. At that time, Mr. Carnegie was a senior citizen and had an insatiable curiosity about the subject of success. He wanted to know: Is there a formula consistent with success? To this end, he commissioned young Napoleon Hill to embark on a twenty-year study. During the study, Mr. Hill was to interview and get to know fifty of the most outstandingly successful people in the world and then determine if there was a common denominator that made them successful.

Some of the people he worked with and studied closely over the twenty-year period were Henry Ford, George Eastman, Theodore Roosevelt, William Jennings Bryan, John D. Rockefeller, Thomas Edison, Woodrow Wilson, William Howard Taft, Alexander Bell, and of course Mr. Carnegie himself. Needless to say, this partial listing includes some of the most successful people the world has ever known.

Napoleon Hill was not the only person to pursue the subject of success in our modern day. Other contemporaries such as Dr. Norman Vincent Peale, Dr. Maxwell Maltz, Dr. Robert Schuller, Claude M. Bristol, W.

Clement Stone, and others have devoted a lifetime to the study of success. They have developed various philosophies—"The Power of Positive Thinking," "Psychocybernetics," "Possibility Thinking," etc. These people have all come to one basic conclusion—your thought process is responsible for your success or lack of it. You become *what* you think about.

You might wonder if the study of the thought process and how it determines success or lack of success is just a modern-day phenomenon. It isn't. Throughout history, numerous observations have been made by some of the great teachers and philosophers.

Disraeli said, "Everything comes if a man will only wait. I have brought myself by long meditation to the conclusion that a person with a settled purpose must accomplish it."

The great Roman emperor Marcus Aurelius once said, "A man's life is what his thoughts make of it."

Ralph Waldo Emerson stated that, "A man is what he thinks about all day long."

Napoleon Hill, in one of his many books wrote, "Whatever the mind of man can conceive and believe, it can achieve."

The British philosopher James Allen wrote a book in 1902 titled *As a Man Thinketh*. In it he states:

> As a man thinketh in his heart, so is he. This embraces the whole of a man's being. It is so comprehensive that it reaches out to every condition and circumstance of life. A man is literally what he thinks. His character is the sum of all his thoughts. Of all the beautiful truths pertaining to the soul, none is more gladdening or fruitful of divine promise and confidence than this—that a man is the master of thought, the molder of character, and the maker and shaper of condition, environment, and his own destiny.

Even though the evidence is overwhelming that there is a relationship between the way you think and your success or lack of same, fewer than 5 percent of the population know about it.

So, what does success have to do with high-level wellness? The answer is really very simple. Turning failure into success—eliminating negative lifestyles—is the path to the high-level wellness you seek. You must understand that *achieving high-level wellness is no different than accomplishing any other significant or important goal in life*. The basic reason the majority fail is that they ignore the thought process.

The most productive form of positive thinking is visualization. You can communicate adequately with your subconscious mind through positive thinking and achieve success in any endeavor, but it is many times more effective if you can transmit your thoughts via mental pictures. *Visualization is the single most important factor in the elimination of negative lifestyles and achieving high-level wellness.*

In the past if you have tried to stop smoking, lose weight, stay on a regular exercise program, eat more nutritious meals, reduce or eliminate alcohol, or learn to cope with stress and failed, you now know the reason why. All the programs, plans, and techniques you have tried failed to recognize that before you can change or alter behavioral patterns, you must first condition the mind.

CONFORMITY AND NONCONFORMITY

It is a paradox that even though we have such magnificent minds we devote such minimal effort to activities such as thinking and visualization. In one of the last interviews he granted, Dr. Albert Schweitzer was asked, "What's wrong with man today?" After serious contemplation, the wise old doctor replied, "Man simply does not think." How true. Have you ever wondered: What's the consequence of not thinking? It's *conformity*.

In the past, many have caused premature aging and premature death because they conformed. It was not popular to examine lifestyles and learn how and why they were harmful. Everyone just assumed that there was nothing which could be done to alter what came down the road of illness, so just conform and be like all the other people. Now you are one of the tens of millions who are becoming a nonconformist, a thinking person, who has decided to take charge of your own health destiny. This is great. Become a nonconformist, not for the sake of being a maverick, but so that you will question your current state of wellness.

Nonconformity is one of the prime reasons for the current Wellness Renaissance which is sweeping the nation. Nonconformity has caused us pioneers of wellness not to be satisfied with the traditional methods of treatment/cure. It has caused us to question and inquire, "Isn't there a better way?"

One of the greatest examples of being a nonconformist I know of is illustrated by Norman Cousins, illustrious former editor of the *Saturday Review*. In 1964, Norman Cousins was diagnosed as having ankylosing spondylitis, which is an extremely painful disease, one in which the spine and other joints of the body literally fuse together. Death is the usual end result. Mr. Cousins was told by his physicians that his chance for recovery was one in five hundred. Being a curious and questioning individual, Mr. Cousins was not willing to accept these odds. He decided he should and would make a major personal contribution to his own medical history.

After Mr. Cousins was informed by his physician of the diagnosis, he remembered reading a book entitled *The Stress of Life* that was published in 1957 by Dr. Hans Selye of Montreal. Dr. Selye is considered today the "father of the study of stress" and what it does to and for people. In the book, Dr. Selye points out that stress leads to distress and distress can cause virtually every medical disease or abnormality known to man. Mr. Cousins' thinking was that if stress can lead to various physical and mental diseases, would it not be true that an environment of happiness, hope, love, faith, and the will to live could reverse disease conditions? So his experiment involved watching, for a number of hours each day, old slapstick movies—the Marx Brothers, Laurel and Hardy, Abbott and Costello type—plus tapes of the television series "Candid Camera." In addition, he was constantly encouraged by family and friends. They insisted he would recover. After devoting hours each day to watching these movies and being in a positive, encouraging environment, Mr. Cousins came to a conclusion. He said that five minutes of hearty laughter resulted in two hours of pain-free time for him. Mr. Cousins did not attempt a scientific explanation for his observation. It was twelve years later that a possible scientific explanation came along, when it was discovered for the first time that the brain secretes a protein-like material called endorphines. We now know that endorphines are at least as potent as morphine in killing pain. When are endorphines elaborated? In response to laughter and a happy attitude. So you see, Norman Cousins, on his own, made a discovery, and that is, your mental attitude does have direct bearing on the control of pain and prognosis of diseases.

In addition to relief of pain, Mr. Cousins also noticed that the environment and attitude which he developed for himself caused a drop in his sedimentation rate. This is a laboratory blood test which determines the presence of infection or inflammation. Ankylosing spondylitis is an inflammatory disease, so through the daily declining sedimentation rate, Mr. Cousins had definite proof that happiness and laughter was curing his disease.

You might be interested in knowing the outcome of Mr. Cousins' condition. He's alive and well today and the author of the best-selling book *The Anatomy of an Illness*. Doctors call it a miracle. Mr. Cousins says it's the psychology of laughter and attitude of mind that cured him.

BEHAVIORAL MEDICINE

So what does this mean? It simply means that your attitude, your temperament, your mood, the way you think, whatever you want to call it, has an active feedback effect on your physical health. The way you think does have a pronounced effect on causing, preventing, or healing diseases. In this modern day and age, in the 1980s, it has come to be referred to as *behavioral medicine.*

Behavioral medicine is defined as treating or preventing diseases by modifying or changing personal behavior and/or lifestyles. Behavioral medicine is taught as a formal subject in a significant number of our medical schools.

This new and exciting discipline of medicine is the result of the blending of psychiatric and biological medicine. As we learn more about the mind and the impact it has on keeping us well or making us sick, the curiosity increases about controlling the thought process to make it work for us instead of against us.

I would like to share with you what James Allen wrote in *As a Man Thinketh* about the relationship between the thought process and health:

> The body is the servant of the mind. It obeys the operations of the mind whether they are deliberately chosen or automatically expressed. At the bidding of unlawful thoughts, the body sinks rapidly into disease and decay. At the command of glad and beautiful thoughts, it becomes clothed with youthfulness and beauty. Disease and health-like circumstances are rooted in thought. Sickly thoughts will express themselves through a sickly body. Thoughts of fear have been known to kill a man just as speedily as a bullet and they are continuing to kill thousands of people just as surely, though less rapidly. The people who live in fear of disease are the people who get it. Anxiety quickly demoralizes the whole body, and lays it open to the entrance of disease. Impure thoughts, even if not physically indulged, soon will shatter the nervous system. Strong, pure, and happy thoughts build up the body in vigor and grace. The body is a delicate and plastic instrument which responds readily to thought, and thought will produce its own effects, good or bad, upon it.
>
> If you would perfect your body, guard your mind. If you would renew your body, beautify your mind.

The body will always respond to the thought process, whether positive or negative. It is important that you understand that the body has no way of determining if thoughts are negative or positive. It will always react according to the thought process. If you are involved in negative thoughts, illness and failure will result. If you are constantly generating positive thoughts, nothing but disease-free and positive things will happen. This is a basic law of nature. It never fails.

THE POWER OF VISUALIZATION

You already know that visualization is the development of and concentration on a specific and detailed mental picture. This is a general definition. Now that you have learned about the relationship between thinking and success, and thinking and visualization, it's time to consider the technique of visualization in greater detail.

Visualization is a highly controlled form of thinking. It's disciplined imagination. Some feel that visualization is simply forming a mental picture. It's much more. Visualization is not only creating a mental picture, but it's *making the picture come alive.* The mental picture must be so vivid that it is *real.* It must have color, depth, sound, smell, and touch. You must actually be able to feel, experience, and become a part of the mental picture just as if it is occurring in your world.

Can you visualize? This may sound like an overly simple question but it isn't. Research has pointed out that individuals have varying degrees of ability to visualize. It is estimated that 15 percent of the population are *visualizers.* They have a tendency to have vivid imaginations and to think in mental pictures. If you are in this group, you already know exactly what I am talking about and know how to visualize. About the same number—15 percent—are *verbalizers.* These are individuals who tend to think with words instead of mental pictures. If you are a verbalizer you may be having serious doubts about the entire subject of visualization, because it could be a new experience for you. There is no question that verbalizers must exert more effort to visualize in a real-life way. The remaining 70 percent are a visualizer-verbalizer combination. They tend to think with mental pictures and words.

Regardless of where you are on the visualizer-verbalizer spectrum, you can learn to become a proficient visualizer. It's a skill that can be learned and perfected.

Napoleon said, "The human race is governed by its imagination." Albert Einstein was of the opinion that "imagination is more important than knowledge." Visualization is imagination brought to life.

The power of visualization can be illustrated in the works of Dr. O. Carl Simonton, who is a cancer specialist. Dr. Simonton has published extensively on the effect of the thought process in curing or altering the progress of cancer. Dr. Simonton, early in his medical training, had a very high curiosity as to why it was that some cancer patients experienced spontaneous remissions from this normally incurable disease. To this extent, Dr. Simonton designed several studies to try to answer this question. First he conducted a retrospective study, in which he identified and obtained the case records of individuals who had experienced bonafide spontaneous remissions from a variety of different types of cancer. After careful study of each case record, he talked with the patients, their families, and their physicians. He wanted to find out if there was any single, common denominator that would set these patients, who had spontaneous remissions, aside from other cancer patients. He found after thorough study and investigation that there was a common denominator. Each of these patients was exceedingly optimistic and was a positive thinker. From the beginning, instead of accepting the fact that cancer is always an incurable disease, they expressed the opinion that they would overcome the problem and be cured of the disease. They knew about the thought process and understood how to utilize it.

After making this important observation, Dr. Simonton decided to design a prospective study. His new study was to include fifty patients with a variety of different types of cancer. All fifty patients were given the appropriate conventional therapy, chemotherapy, radiotherapy, or that which was indicated. Then Dr. Simonton introduced a new concept—the concept of VISUALIZATION. Dr. Simonton operated under the assumption that all of us have cancer cells in our body at different times during our lifetime. The reason we do not become symptomatic is because our immune system controls cancer cell reproduction and prevents growth and spread of the disease. For the patients in his study, he developed a laymen's course in immunology in which he used a variety of diagrams to illustrate for the cancer patients what a cancer cell looks like, what their immune system looks like, and how it looks when attacking cancer cells and killing them. He then had diagrams illustrating what the immune system looks like carrying dead cancer cells away. These patients, after studying this system and technique, were instructed to visualize their own body killing and carrying away dead cancer cells. They practiced this visualization technique three times each day.

According to statistics, approximately 1 to 2 percent of all cancer patients experience spontaneous remissions of the disease. From this standpoint, Dr. Simonton would have expected either none or, at best, one of his fifty patients to have a spontaneous remission. After going through the conventional therapy, receiving strong reinforcement and practicing visualization techniques, twelve of the fifty had what was judged to be excellent regressions of their tumors. Based on preliminary evaluation, eight of the twelve had been given less than a fifty-fifty chance of improvement.

The process of visualization is a major breakthrough. It is an organized system of mind control which can cause the cure of diseases or the modification of a disease process.

Increasing studies of this type are appearing in medical literature. Much still needs to be done, and it will be, but the data which exists is clear. We have contained within ourselves powerful, controllable factors which can keep us well, make us ill, or cure us after we become sick.

Visualization is exciting, dynamic and it works. This program for high-level wellness, which you are going to learn about, is the first to use visualization for behavorial modification and lifestyle change. By using this technique, no negative lifestyle is too resistant or stubborn for removal from your life forever.

THE PLAN FOR THE ELIMINATION OF NEGATIVE LIFESTYLES

By way of review, the two most important factors involved in achieving high-level wellness and living longer and feeling better are:

- realization and acceptance of wellness self-responsibility
- elimination of all negative lifestyles

It is assumed that you have already accepted a certain degree of wellness self-responsibility or you wouldn't be reading this book. Only you know the commitment you have. Unless it is complete, you must diligently apply yourself until wellness self-responsibility is one of the most important commitments of your life.

The second major factor is the elimination of all negative lifestyles. High-level wellness and negative lifestyles cannot exist together in the same body. Visualization, if applied correctly, never fails in achieving this goal. You must become an expert in converting positive thinking into mental pictures.

How do we go about eliminating our negative lifestyles? First, you must realize that most people have more than one. One of the prime reasons why many people fail when attempting to eliminate them is that they become so enthusiastic they want to eliminate all of them at once. This will not work.

Many of the authorities of thought control have pointed out that the mind responds best to only one suggestion at a time. For this reason, I want you to first establish your own list of priorities for elimination. In order to help you, I have surveyed physicians and experts in the health care field to try to determine what should be the priority for elimination if an individual has all six negative lifestyles. This survey is merely a consensus of opinion, based on a cross section of recommendations.

Priority for the Elimination of Negative Lifestyles

1. Smoking
2. Lack of regular exercise
3. Obesity
4. Inability to cope with everyday stress
5. Poor nutrition
6. Excessive consumption of alcohol

This list makes practical sense. Smoking is at the top of the list because the relationship between smoking, lung cancer, cardiovascular diseases, and premature death is unquestioned. A program for regular sustained exercise makes sense for the second priority not only because of the positive effect on the cardiopulmonary system, but also for the indirect effect it has on the elimination of other negative lifestyles. For example, when individuals go from a sedentary life to one of regular exercise, often they lose weight and find that exercise is the best possible control for everyday stress. The obesity epidemic in the United States must be brought under control. Some feel obesity is the number one cause of premature death. All of us are constantly surrounded by stress. Understanding and developing methods to control stress are essential. We are eating ourselves to death. Remember, you can be malnourished with a full stomach. Malnourishment is involved not only with starvation, but also with eating too much and eating the wrong kinds of food. Consumption of excessive amounts of alcohol is a major problem for many. Just because it is last on the list should not detract from its importance. For some, the elimination or control of alcohol should be first.

It is important to remember that this list is a consensus of opinion. It may not be correct for you. Your job is to think through your priorities, then establish your own personal list for elimination.

Below is a summary of your Plan for the Elimination of Negative Lifestyles. Following the summary is a more in-depth description of the program and explanation of how to make it come alive for you. What you are about to learn could change your entire life. If followed closely, you are about to begin one of the most significant projects of your life, a project that will result in maximizing your life-span and enhancing the quality of your life. You will feel better and live longer.

Step One: Write a list of your negative lifestyles according to your priority for elimination.

Step Two: Select your number one negative lifestyle for elimination.

Step Three: Study and review the chapter in this book that pertains to the negative lifestyle you want to eliminate.

Step Four: Write a summary of everything you learn about how and why your negative lifestyle is affecting your health and body systems. Remember, great mental power is generated when you turn information into knowledge.

Step Five: Develop the ability to mentally visualize how your negative lifestyle is affecting your health and body systems.

Step Six: Practice visualization every morning upon waking, noon, evening, and just before going to sleep. Visualize every time there is an urge to practice the negative lifestyle.

Step Seven: Determine and write down a schedule or target date whereby your negative lifestyle will be eliminated.

Step Eight: Develop a vivid mental image of you without your negative lifestyle.

This simple Plan will allow you to turn failure into success. It doesn't matter what you are working to eliminate. Nor does it matter how many times you have tried and failed. This Plan works every time. All you need to do is apply the methods without deviation and with enthusiasm.

Now that you have reviewed the summary for your Plan for the Elimination of Negative Lifestyles and know how to achieve high-level wellness, I would like to elaborate on each step of the program.

Step One

Write a list of your negative lifestyles according to your priority for elimination. After reading this book and careful evaluation, establish your list of priorities. Think through this exercise carefully. Which of your negative lifestyles do you most want to eliminate? Which is next? And so on. After you have made your decisions, *write* down your list. It is absolutely essential that you write your list. By so doing, you are making a commitment to yourself. In addition, the subconscious mind will always react more strongly to a commitment that is written than one that is not.

Step Two

Select your number one negative lifestyle for elimination. One of the paradoxical facets of wellness is that many people, after realizing the necessity for elimination of negative lifestyles, want to start on a program to eliminate all of them at the same time. *This is a prime reason for failure.* The mind has tremendous influence over the body. However, it can exhibit its maximum influence only when the objective is singular and clearly defined. For this reason, *you must concentrate on the elimination of only one negative lifestyle at a time.* It is essential that you operate as if you have only one negative lifestyle. That's the one at the top of your list. Devote total concentration and effort to its elimination and you will be amazed how easy it is to erase. After you have eliminated the first, full and complete attention may be given to the second. But don't think about the second for now.

Step Three

Study and review the chapter in this book that pertains to the negative lifestyle you want to eliminate. This step in your program is one of the most important. Remember, one of the reasons you do not have sufficient self-responsibility for high-level wellness is because of lack of information and knowledge. You must become your own expert on exactly how and why your negative lifestyle is affecting you and your body systems. This is the basis upon which the entire program works. Study the chapter in Book Two of this book which describes the lifestyle you are eliminating. Turn the information into personal knowledge for yourself. Study the diagrams and artists' concepts of exactly what happens to your vital organs and body systems as you indulge in your negative lifestyle. Go to your library, if you like, to read and study other material. Saturate your brain. Learn *how* and *why* your negative lifestyle will prevent you from living a healthy and longer life.

Step Four

Write a summary of everything you learn about how and why your negative lifestyle is affecting your health and your body systems. As you are learning, take notes. All of us learn faster and retain more if we utilize as many of our senses as possible. After you have learned all you can and are able to personally apply your new knowledge to yourself, write a detailed summary. Remember, information is not powerful until it is turned into knowledge. Then your own subconscious mind will help you achieve maximum wellness.

Step Five

Develop the ability to mentally visualize how your negative lifestyle is affecting your health and body systems. You must develop in your mind a vivid mental picture of how your negative lifestyle affects individual vital organs and body systems. Numerous artists' concepts are provided which illustrate normal functioning body organs and systems. Along with these are illustrations showing the effect of the negative lifestyle. Study the illustrations so you can mentally visualize your negative lifestyle specifically working in the ways it affects body systems. Visualize in great detail. Develop the ability to instantly recall every aspect of what is happening. After studying the illustrations in this book, feel free to develop your own drawings of how the negative lifestyle is harmful to your vital organs and body systems. Anatomical correctness is not important, your involvement is. The more personally involved you become with visualization, the greater its effectiveness.

Step Six

Practice visualization every morning upon waking, noon, evening, and just before going to sleep. Visualize every time there is an urge to practice the negative lifestyle. It is essential that you develop your level of knowledge and implant in your mind the pictures of exactly how and why negative lifestyles are harmful to you. You must have a definite, disciplined schedule for complete recall of all you have learned. By visualizing immediately upon awaking, the tone is set for the day. By having other predetermined times for visualization, it becomes habit and that's what you want. Set your own times. They can be, for instance, at break time, or before, or after, lunch or dinner. Whatever the times, the main point is that you do it every day. Visualization just before going to sleep is probably the most effective, because the subconscious mind can absorb and function during sleep. Get into the habit—every time there is an urge to practice the negative lifestyle—of visualizing. Get a vivid mental picture of exactly how and why the negative lifestyle in which you are about to indulge destroys your vital organs and body systems. Visualization is the key to your program. It will eliminate your negative lifestyle.

Step Seven

Determine and write down a schedule or target date whereby your negative lifestyle will be eliminated. You must have a well-defined goal to work toward. This goal is a definite time or date when the negative lifestyle will be completely eliminated. Without this goal, the mind has nothing to strive for and, therefore, nothing will be accomplished. Goal-setting is a commitment. Any time a commitment exists, the effort expended goes up accordingly.

Step Eight

Develop a vivid mental image of you without your negative lifestyle. Right from the beginning, picture yourself in your mind without your negative lifestyle. For example, if you smoke, get the image of yourself without a cigarette in your hands or mouth, without the bulge in your pocket made by the pack. Imagine not wondering if there are enough cigarettes in the pack to last the evening. Think what it is like without the taste of tobacco smoke in your mouth. Picture what you are going to do with the money you save from not smoking.

If you have not been successful in getting started and staying on a program for regular exercise, develop a picture of yourself in prime physical condition performing your chosen exercise. If your exercise is jogging, picture yourself running five miles or perhaps running and winning a 10,000-meter race. Get a picture of your body not with flabby fat hanging on, but lean and firm. Picture yourself being able to run up four flights of steps without breathing hard. Imagine the pride and self-satisfaction involved with the elimination of a sedentary life.

Other examples could be given. The main point is for you to develop the habit of thinking success. Picture yourself having already achieved your goal.

Well, there you have it—a technique that will make eliminating negative lifestyles easy. Does it sound complex? Perhaps so, but remember that any worthwhile goal in life requires discipline and commitment. This is no different.

WHY IT WORKS

If you haven't already, you should ask why am I so sure this Plan will work for you. The body is like a magnificent machine. It is made up of a series of checks and balances. These checks and balances, which keep you alive and functioning, can be thought of as regulators not unlike the thermostat that turns the furnace on and off. For example, when you become hot the body's thermostats change and you start to perspire, which helps cool the body. When you are cold, the body's thermostats change and you shiver, which helps you warm up. These internal thermostat changes are important in keeping your body temperature at exactly 98.6° F. When you eat a large meal, substantial amounts of glucose (sugar) are taken in. In order to keep the blood sugar within narrow limits, the regulator on your pancreas readjusts and causes insulin to be released, which removes excess glucose from the blood. If you skip a meal or two and the body needs energy, the regulator on the liver changes and releases stored glycogen, which is converted into glucose. When you exercise, the muscles of the body require more oxygen. The regulators readjust, which speeds up breathing and heart rate, so more oxygen is brought in and delivered to the muscles. Dozens of additional examples could be given. Over the years, we have learned a great deal about how well the body adjusts, depending upon external and internal needs.

All of these body changes are initiated by the brain. They are caused by feedback mechanisms. In other words, the brain gets the message that something is not normal, that something has changed or is about to change. As soon as the brain receives this information, the appropriate body systems are called into action by the mind. The mind is totally educated and conditioned to recognize and initiate all required action.

Now—you are probably wondering what this has to do with the elimination of negative lifestyles. *Negative lifestyles are either accepted or rejected based upon signals sent to the body by the mind.* This is the reason why the thought process and visualization must be used if negative lifestyles are to be eliminated.

As James Allen said, "The body is the servant of the mind." The body always reacts to signals from the mind. The mind will always warn the body when it is exposed to or involved in some potentially harmful internal or external activity. The body can't think. It always reacts in accordance with instructions from the mind. The mind issues instruction based upon knowledge. Herein lies the reason why you have negative lifestyles and have failed to eliminate them.

Your mind is not educated about how a negative lifestyle destroys your vital organs and body systems. Therefore, your body accepts and tolerates the negative lifestyle because the mind cannot warn it of the lethal consequences. Thus, your regulators are set to accept negative lifestyles.

The Plan for the Elimination of Negative Lifestyles outlined in this book is designed to eliminate this problem. Your Plan allows your mind to become completely informed and educated as to exactly *how* and *why* your negative lifestyle detracts from longevity and high-quality life. *How* and *why* vital organs and body systems are destroyed. Once the mind fully comprehends and understands the dire personal consequences of multinegative lifestyles, new and appropriate signals are automatically sent to the body. Based upon these new warning signals, the various regulators of the body readjust, making the negative lifestyle *totally unacceptable and, therefore, rejected.*

You might wonder what is the end result of this program. Individuals who have attended Wellness Seminars often report the following:

- Smoking becomes distasteful, for some to the point of nausea.
- Those who are overweight report a dramatic decrease in appetite.
- Foods which are known to be harmful become unpalatable.
- Many report more interest in the "smaller things" of life and find it easier to relax.
- Lack of regular, sustained exercise results in a feeling of guilt.
- Consumption of alcohol is eliminated or reduced because of a lack of desire for the intoxicated feeling.

Why do these dramatic, almost unbelievable, changes take place? Some say it's self-hypnosis. Others feel it's autosuggestion. These may seem like logical explanations, but they are not true. The fact is, for the first time you have implanted in your thought process information which describes the consequences of negative lifestyles. The mind finally understands why premature death occurs. Once this happens, the mind informs the body that negative lifestyles are no longer acceptable and therefore are not tolerated. Feeling better and living longer is at last a reality.

You may wonder: Is it worth the effort? Remember, the end result of high-level wellness is maximum life-span, highest-quality life, increased ambition and productivity, greater self-satisfaction and self-esteem. I am talking about changes that can make you a new and better person. Today is the day to start your life of high-level wellness.

You have now finished Book One. It is designed to educate and instruct you in the system for achieving high-level wellness through the elimination of negative lifestyles. It also explains how and why the system works.

Book Two is actually six books in one. There is a chapter devoted to the elimination of each of the six negative lifestyles plus a brief chapter about the future for wellness. The chapters are titled:

- Yes, You Can Stop Smoking!
- Coping with Everyday Stress
- How to Eat, Drink, and Be Healthy
- How to Get Your Weight Down Starting Now!
- How to Moderate Your Drinking—or Quit Completely If You Wish
- Physical Fitness, Today, Tomorrow, and Forever
- Your Future Full of Wellness

By now you should have established your list of priority for the elimination of your negative lifestyles. If you have not, do so at this time. You should then proceed directly to that chapter devoted to the negative lifestyle which tops your list. The question comes up frequently, "Can't I read the entire book before deciding which negative lifestyle I want to eliminate first?" If you like, go ahead, but it is imperative that you don't start your program if you are going to take this route. After you have read all of Book Two, then return to the chapter involved with the negative lifestyle you are going to eliminate. Reread and study it in detail. Put all the other chapters out of your mind. Total concentration and visualization must be directed toward the negative lifestyle you are about to eliminate forever. After this negative lifestyle is gone, proceed to the chapter concerned with your second for elimination. After this has been accomplished, go to the third. Continue until all negative lifestyles are eliminated and you are standing at the pinnacle of wellness. Then you will realize the ultimate human experience, maximum life-span and enhanced quality of life. This seemed impossible a short while ago, but not now, because you are USING VISUALIZATION AND THE THOUGHT PROCESS TO FEEL BETTER AND LIVE LONGER.

BOOK TWO

4. YES, YOU CAN STOP SMOKING!

"You don't mind if I smoke, do you?"
"Not if you don't mind my being sick."

If you are a smoker and for some reason don't want to stop smoking read no further. I say this because some people do not really want to stop. So, be sure of your intentions and real desires, because after you have read this chapter and apply the program as prescribed, you will have no choice. You will stop smoking. The thing you will find strange is that you will stop smoking with no conscious effort. So, regardless of how many times you have tried to quit and failed, regardless of how long you have smoked or the number of cigarettes smoked per day, you are, at this moment, beginning your personal countdown to becoming an ex-smoker.

Smoking is one of the most dangerous of our negative lifestyles. Fifty million people smoke. The incidence of smoking among men is on a downward trend. So is lung cancer. The trend among teenagers is increasing at about the same rate it is decreasing among men. Thus, among these two groups, smoking remains about constant.

Recently a report from the Surgeon General of the United States pointed out that 30 percent of American women are smoking. Smoking among American women is increasing so rapidly that by the year 1983, cancer of the lung in American women will surpass cancer of the breast to become the most prevalent malignancy among women.

I want to remind you that one of the prime reasons you have not been able to quit smoking is because, although you may not realize it, you lack self-responsibility. Or rather, what you lack is the information and knowledge that will enable you to take that responsibility. This chapter will give you all the tools you will need.

In order for you to quit smoking you need to understand exactly *how* and *why* smoking affects you. This information is utilized in the Plan for Elimination of Negative Lifestyles. Once you thoroughly absorb what it really means to smoke, your untapped impulses will gain significant power and your own body will reject smoking.

Let's stop for a moment and briefly review our system for Elimination of Negative Lifestyles. In summary, the system involves visualization. First, from the material you learn in this chapter and other reference sources, become an expert on exactly *how* and *why* smoking affects you. As you are learning, write a summary of exactly *how* and *why* smoking is harmful to you. Develop the ability to mentally visualize exactly *how* smoking is harmful to each of your vital organs and body systems. Discipline yourself to visualize these harmful actions taking place as soon as you wake, several times during the morning, afternoon, evening, and the last thing before you go to sleep. Also develop the automatic response to "visualize" every time you have the urge to smoke or each time you light up.

Next, you must select a date when you no longer will smoke, or a schedule whereby you will reduce the number of cigarettes smoked each day. Be sure you write your goal down along with your written summary of *how* and *why* smoking affects vital organs and body systems. Lastly, *develop the mental picture of yourself without cigarettes*. Think of all the benefits you will derive from not smoking—longer life, feeling better with greater energy, saving money, not being a bother to others who are nonsmokers and not being a slave to an addicting habit. Remember, this system works every time. It takes time and effort, but any goal worth achieving is worth working for.

So with this brief review, we are ready to start your program. You are about to become an expert on the subject of smoking.

SMOKING

When tobacco is burned, hundreds of identifiable chemical compounds are given off. It would serve no purpose to list all of them, but a few of the more interesting ones are: carbon monoxide, nicotine, hydrogen cyanide, arsenic trioxide, and tars.

Tobacco Tar and Cancer

Tobacco tar is a carcinogen. It causes cancer in both animals and humans. So much has been written proving the cause-effect relationship between tobacco tar and lung cancer that it needs no further elaboration. It is necessary to point out that lung cancer is usually an extremely painful and undignified way to die. It has been estimated that if all smoking ceased, cases of lung cancer would decrease by 90 percent and deaths due to lung cancer would drop 80 percent.

The question always arises why some people smoke for many years and never develop lung cancer while others do. It could be involved in the individual's own natural defense system. Perhaps some have a more highly developed and resistant immune system. There is genetic research being conducted about this now. Other factors include how young the individual was when he or she started smoking, how long the individual has smoked, how many cigarettes smoked per day, and how far down the cigarette is routinely smoked. If the cigarette is not smoked beyond half of its length, the tobacco itself acts as a filter and tends to diminish the amount of tar and nicotine that is taken into the lungs. All of these are important factors.

While the association between smoking and lung cancer is well-known, the relationship between smoking and other types of cancer is less publicized and understood.

There is a direct relation between smoking and an increase of cancer of the mouth, pharynx, larynx, and esophagus. The possibility of these cancers seems to increase even further if the individual drinks alcohol on a regular basis. Chronic alcohol consumption may remove the "protective barrier" from the mouth and throat which makes it easier for cancer to develop.

Smoking increases the possibility of cancer of the bladder. Tobacco tar which is taken in through the lungs, then transferred into the blood, is excreted mainly through the urine. In some cases, the tobacco tar residue can be retained in the bladder up to ten hours. This unnatural concentration of tobacco tar in the urine, which is retained in the bladder, is the prime reason for the increase in bladder cancer among smokers.

When considering all forms of cancer, the *Surgeon General's Report* points out, *"Cigarette smokers are about twice as likely to die of cancer as nonsmokers."* Do you comprehend what this means? By smoking, you are *doubling* your chances of developing a terminal case of cancer. Is it really worth it?

What you must do is become totally informed about the cancer-causing properties of tobacco tar and understand that cancer is something that does not always happen to the other person. It can strike you. By stopping the smoking habit, you become actively involved in reducing your chances of developing one of our most dreaded diseases.

Nicotine

Nicotine is a powerful and potent drug. Fortunately there are only minute quantities found in tobacco. It has been estimated that five drops of pure nicotine would be a lethal dose for the average human. When nicotine is inhaled into the lungs via tobacco smoke, it is quickly transferred into the blood.

Once in the circulatory system, nicotine causes a sharp increase in the secretion of epinephrine (adrenaline). Epinephrine causes several things to happen. First, it is a potent cardiac agent and as such causes an increase in heart rate. Second, it is a vasoconstrictor, which means it causes the arteries to constrict and thus increase the blood pressure.

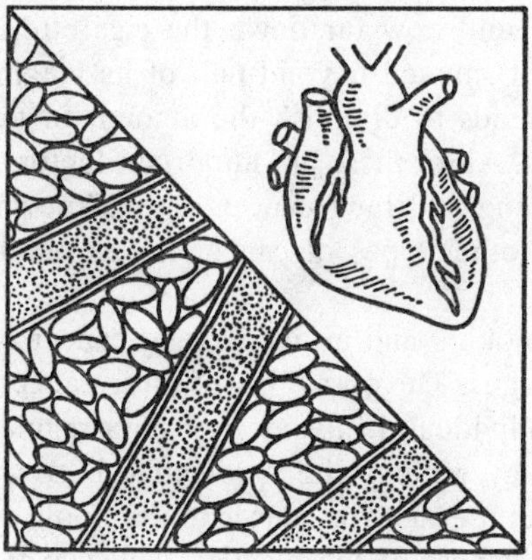

Nonsmoker: The arteries are not constricted and the heart rate is normal.

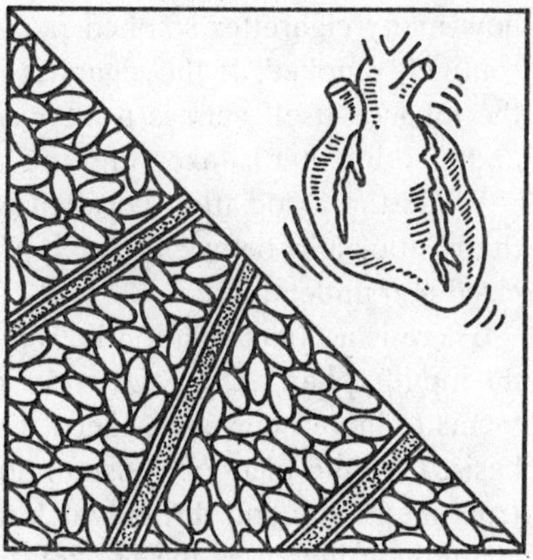

Nicotine effect: The arteries are constricted, the blood pressure is up, and the heart rate is increased.

For most people, taking a drug which causes the heart to race or the blood pressure to go up is not good. Yet every time you light up, inhale your nicotine, it happens. Can you imagine the results when nicotine is ingested by a person who has a history of heart problems or already has high blood pressure? Does it now make sense that most physicians recommend that cardiac or hypertensive (high blood pressure) patients stop smoking?

Carbon Monoxide (CO)

Over the years, most of the attention to the harmful effects of smoking has been directed toward research and study of tars and nicotine. This has been good in that we have a good working knowledge of how the various vital organs and body systems react to constant insult by these foreign substances.

But more recently, increased emphasis is being directed toward the carbon monoxide (CO) content of tobacco and its effect on various body systems. As has been pointed out, CO is one of the hundred or so chemical compounds given off when tobacco is burned. CO wreaks its damage primarily on the blood system.

Blood is made up of several formed elements. One of these is the red blood cells. Contained within the red blood cells is hemoglobin. One of the prime functions of hemoglobin is to pick up and transport oxygen from the lungs throughout the body. It is also responsible for picking up carbon dioxide from the body and releasing it through the lungs by exhalation.

The main problem is that hemoglobin is not loyal to oxygen. It can and will pick up a variety of other items when available. One compound which hemoglobin loves more than oxygen is carbon monoxide. The affinity of CO for hemoglobin is about two hundred times greater than the attraction of oxygen for hemoglobin. Usually this presents no problem because normally we have only trace amounts of CO in the blood. However, when tobacco smoke is inhaled, the CO in the blood goes up quickly and significantly. Since the love affair between hemoglobin and CO is deeper than that between hemoglobin and oxygen, the CO quickly attaches itself to the hemoglobin. The load which hemoglobin can carry (CO or oxygen) is limited. For this reason, when higher concentrations of CO are in the blood, it attaches itself to the hemoglobin, preventing the attachment of oxygen. This entire process is pictured in the following illustration.

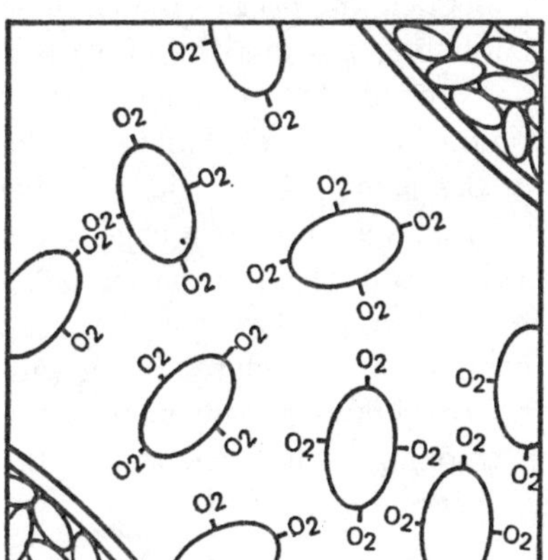

Nonsmoker: The hemoglobin is carrying the maximum amount of oxygen to the body tissues. The blood is oxygen-rich.

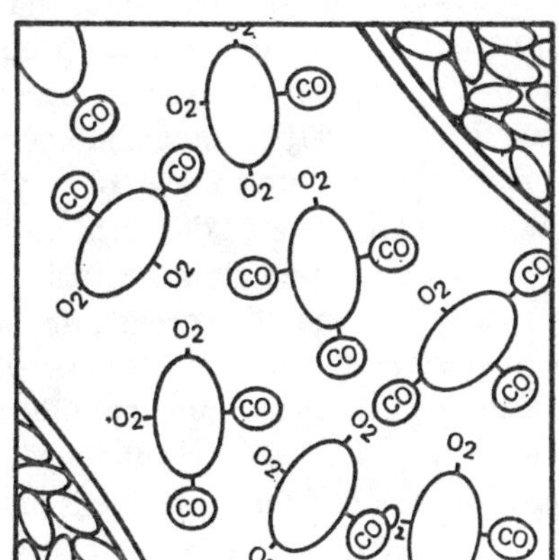

Smoker: Carbon monoxide (CO) has blocked the oxygen's ability to attach to the hemoglobin. The blood is oxygen-starved.

The diagram to the left shows the oxygen-rich hemoglobin of a nonsmoker. To the right is the oxygen-starved blood of a smoker. You can see how the CO has attached itself, preventing a normal load of oxygen from being carried to the cells and tissues of the body.

This oxygen-reduced blood, caused by smoking, has a number of subtle and devastating effects on vital organs and body systems. First is the brain. Smokers deprive the brain of oxygen which is required for its normal function and maintenance. Every cell of the body requires oxygen for normal metabolism and reproduction. This reduction in available oxygen explains why smokers get tired more quickly, are listless, and have less energy than nonsmokers. Also, since less oxygen is available to be carried to the surface of the body and the skin, smokers tend to have a pale and sallow complexion.

It is important for you to have a good working understanding of how carbon monoxide inhaled while smoking reduces the oxygen available to the body. Develop the ability to visualize your hemoglobin and the action of CO against it. Know why, as a smoker, you have less energy and get tired more quickly. Realize you are depriving the brain of needed oxygen. Understand why you have taken some of the blush and beauty from your complexion.

Each year approximately ten thousand people die from carbon monoxide poisoning. You've heard the tragic story. The automobile is started in the garage with the door shut. Within a brief period someone is found dead on the floor. Why do people die so quickly from carbon monoxide poisoning?

When an internal combustion engine is operated, the prime exhaust fume is carbon monoxide. Without proper ventilation, the amount of carbon monoxide in the atmosphere becomes very concentrated. When this is breathed, the carbon monoxide concentration in the blood builds rapidly and blocks the attachment of oxygen to the hemoglobin. With massive doses of carbon monoxide such as you get from an automobile engine, the blockage of oxygen from hemoglobin accelerates until no oxygen is being transported. When this occurs, the brain dies. The point I'm trying to make is that when someone smokes, or when someone is in a closed room with an automobile engine running, precisely the same thing is happening to the blood system. The only difference about smoking a cigarette, is that the total dose of carbon monoxide is much smaller and controlled.

The Platelets

There is yet another major harmful effect of smoking on the blood system. This involves the platelets. When you cut yourself, the platelets are active in causing the blood to clot, thereby preventing profuse bleeding.

Normally, the platelets are well distributed throughout the blood and flow easily throughout the body. Smoking causes the platelets to clump together. This is illustrated in the following drawing:

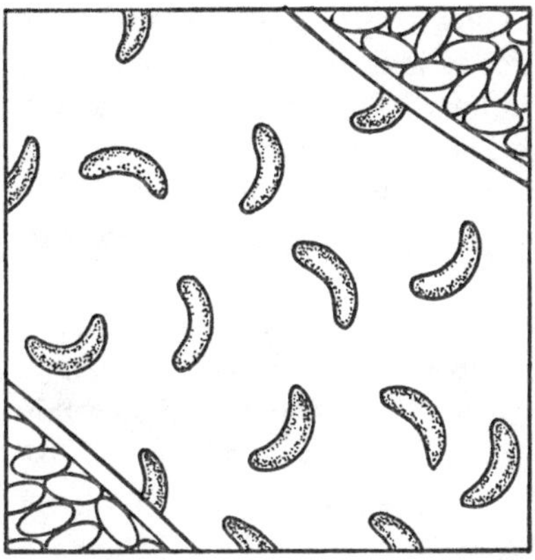

Nonsmoker: The platelets are moving freely in the blood.

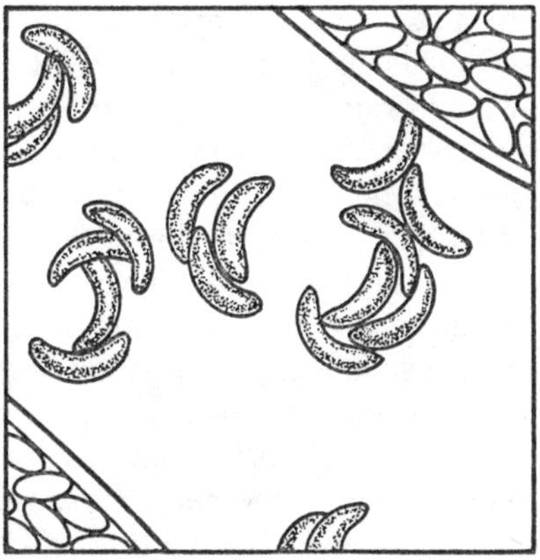

Smoker: The platelets are clumping together, reducing the blood flow.

In the diagram on the left, the platelets can be seen flowing in a well-distributed fashion. This is a nonsmoker.

On the right is the clumping phenomenon, which occurs to smokers. The platelets physically clump together. As this occurs, blood flow is reduced. Blood flow at the capillary level may be reduced significantly by the clumping of smokers' platelets. The problem presented by this reduced blood flow is twofold. First, as blood flow slows, the possibility for intravascular clotting (development of a blood clot within a blood vessel) increases. If clots form and then break off and lodge in the brain, heart, or lungs, serious medical problems result. Second, the reduced blood flow adds further to the problem of reduced oxygen distribution to the cells and tissue of the body.

Cardiovascular Diseases

It has been estimated by the American Heart Association that smokers have a 3.6 times greater chance of developing cardiovascular diseases than nonsmokers and, in fact, a two times greater chance of a heart attack. You don't have to be a professional gambler to recognize that these odds are not in your favor. Keep in mind, you are gambling here with a potential life or death situation. But in spite of the overwhelmingly unfavorable odds, millions continue to smoke. Why? It is because smokers may have the general notion that smoking is not good for you, but, until now, have lacked the specific information and knowledge about exactly *how* and *why* smoking destroys vital organs and body systems.

As a smoker, it is important for you to know why your chances for cardiovascular diseases are higher. I have already indicated that nicotine is a powerful drug, which causes an increase in heart rate. The heart muscle is no different than any other muscle in the body. The harder it works, the more oxygen it must have. But a paradox is involved. You already know that because of the carbon monoxide and platelet clumping, oxygen supply is diminished. So we have a situation where, because of smoking, the heart muscle says, "I need more oxygen," yet subnormal amounts of oxygen are available. This situation is referred to as *myocardial insufficiency*. The heart muscle is demanding more oxygen than it can get. Under this condition, muscle tissue can deteriorate. Thus, the reduced amount of oxygen available to the heart muscle can lead to conditions such as angina (chest pain) and a heart attack.

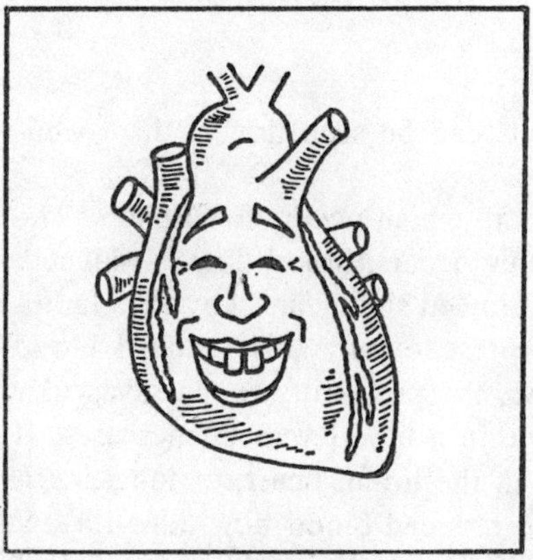

Happy heart: A nonsmoker with sufficient oxygen for the heart muscle.

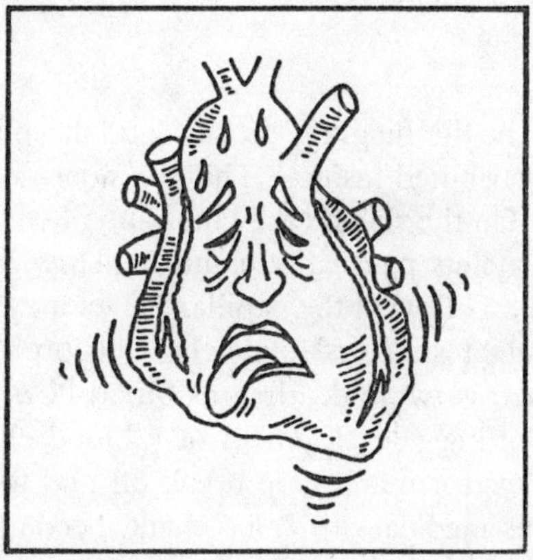

Myocardial insufficiency: Nicotine causes increased work. The carbon monoxide reduces needed oxygen.

The above is an attempt to provide you with a visual image of what myocardial insufficiency is all about. You must think about your heart and the paradox you create in regard to the heart's oxygen demand-supply situation each time you light up.

Statistically speaking, smokers have a much greater chance of stroke, because the nicotine causes hypertension (high blood pressure). Since the blood is moving through the arteries at increased pressure, there is a possibility of bursting a blood vessel. When this occurs with a brain artery, part of the brain is deprived of blood and a portion dies from lack of oxygen. Many are familiar with the end results of a cerebral stroke—death, paralysis, loss of speech or other motor functions. Intravascular clots which result from platelet clumping can also provide major problems. After blood clots form within the blood vessels, they may break loose and travel to different parts of the body. If the traveling clot lodges in a brain artery, it is called a *cerebral embolism.* The clot stops blood flow and a portion of the brain dies. The end result is a stroke. Sometimes, the clot may lodge in one of the main arteries of the lung or heart. Again, there is lack of blood flow and tissue dies. These conditions are referred to as a *pulmonary embolism* and a *coronary embolism.* This could mean loss of lung function or a heart attack.

You must develop the ability to visualize what the platelet system looks like. Develop a vivid mental picture of how the platelets circulate freely and uninhibited in the nonsmoker. Then get a mental picture of your inhibited, clumping platelets under the influence of your habit. Understand how this could lead to a clot and reduce oxygen circulation to your body.

Bronchopulmonary Diseases

The human lung is a magnificent organ. Through the generations and centuries, it has acclimated to inhaling and expelling a variety of foreign materials and substances. This is accomplished through the activity of the cilia, which are tiny hair-like fibers which line the bronchial tubes. The cilia move constantly in a wave-like fashion and push and move dust and foreign particles out of the bronchial tubes. Mucus is secreted within the bronchial tubes in order to facilitate the removal of the foreign particles.

The problem with smoking is, once again, nicotine. Nicotine has an anesthetizing effect on the cilia, rendering them immobile. When a person starts smoking, this effect on the cilia is temporary. However, smoking over a period of years causes the cilia to become permanently anesthetized with loss of function. Foreign particles and mucus accumulate in the bronchial tubes. This unnatural accumulation leads to irritation which is called *chronic bronchitis.* In smokers, the incidence of chronic bronchitis is six times greater than in the nonsmoker.

Everyone is familiar with "smoker's cough." If you don't have it yet and continue to smoke, you will. The increase in cough reflex is in recognition of foreign particle and mucus accumulation due to lost cilia function. The body's own natural method for removing foreign particles and mucus is diminished or lost. In this case, the cough mechanism is substituted. Coughing is a poor substitute for cilia function, but for the long-term smoker, it's the only thing left.

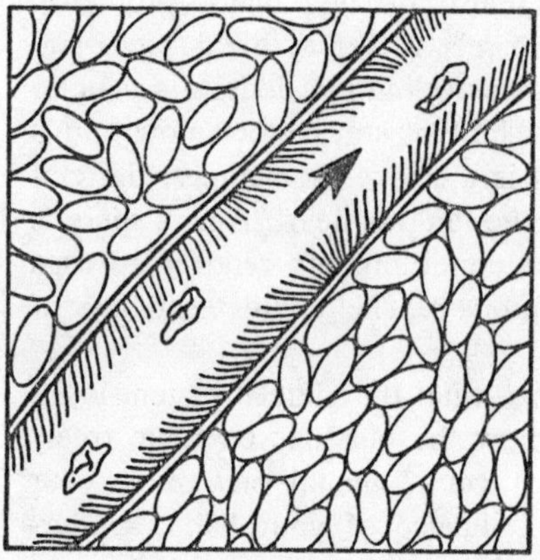

Nonsmoker: Healthy, functioning lung cilia, efficiently moving foreign particles and mucus out of a bronchial tube.

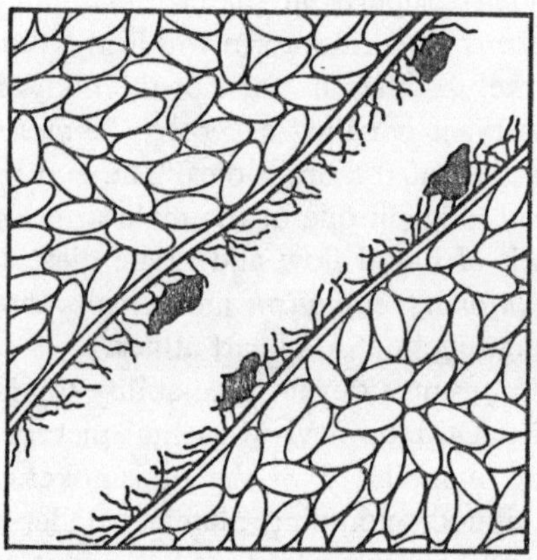

Smoker's lung cilia: Completely anesthetized, with foreign particles and mucus accumulating in a bronchial tube.

Emphysema is one of the most debilitating lung diseases which can be caused by smoking. The main function of a lung is to deliver oxygen to the blood so that it can be distributed throughout the body. It is also responsible for removing carbon dioxide from the blood. These activities are accomplished by tiny sac-like structures in the lungs called alveolar sacs. There are hundreds of these tiny air sacs in each lung. In some way which is not clearly understood, smoking destroys the alveolar sacs. Some think that smoking interrupts the blood flow to the alveolar sacs, thus causing their destruction. Others are of the opinion that they are destroyed as a direct result of one or more of the chemical compounds that are in tobacco smoke.

Regardless, the end result of emphysema is a marked reduction in the capability of the lungs to release oxygen into the blood and expel carbon dioxide. This means that the person with emphysema must breathe much more often just to deliver minimal amounts of oxygen to the body.

A person with healthy lungs will inhale and exhale about fifteen times per minute. A person with emphysema must breathe twenty-five to thirty times per minute. It has been estimated that an individual with healthy lungs expends approximately 5 percent of body energy for breathing. The emphysemic person will use as much as *80 percent of total body energy just for breathing.* Emphysema causes a person to suffocate even though they are breathing as hard as possible. The chances for a smoker to develop emphysema are six to seven times greater than for a nonsmoker.

It is imperative that you develop the ability to mentally visualize the effects of smoking on your lungs. Look at the previous illustration. Each time you light a cigarette or have the urge to smoke, allow the picture to flash across your mind of those anesthetized cilia and the accumulation of all kinds of foreign particles and mucus. Picture the exchange of oxygen and carbon dioxide being significantly diminished. Project the image of why you have smoker's cough. Try to get the feel of labored breathing. You must become your own personal expert on *how* and *why* smoking causes bronchopulmonary diseases.

Brain Function and Smoking

Sometimes during Wellness Seminars an experiment is conducted which illustrates the effect of smoking on brain function. This is an extremely easy experiment. All we need is an electroencephalograph, which is a machine used to measure brain waves. The electrodes are attached to the skull in a prescribed manner. As was pointed out in the previous chapter, each of us is transmitting brain waves at all times. For this reason, we can immediately pick up the brain waves of our subject. At the same time, we can determine the electrical output of the brain.

The next step is to get the subject who is being monitored to light up and inhale deeply several times. The results are amazing. The electrical output of the brain is depressed significantly, sometimes by as much as 50 percent! In addition, alpha wave transmission is usually speeded up and converted to beta waves. Alpha waves are an indication of a relaxed but alert mind. Beta waves are characteristic of mental agitation.

This is visual proof that smoking affects the brain. Now, what's happening? The reduction in the electrical activity of the brain and the increase in brain wave speed may be caused by the increase in secretion of epinephrine and decrease in oxygen supply to the brain. Simply put, it is physiologically bad for you to reduce the electrical activity of the brain and increase brain wave speed.

The two following diagrams represent what a typical experiment of this type might show. On the left is a normal electroencephalogram (EEG). On the right is the EEG of the same person while smoking. It is easy to see the change.

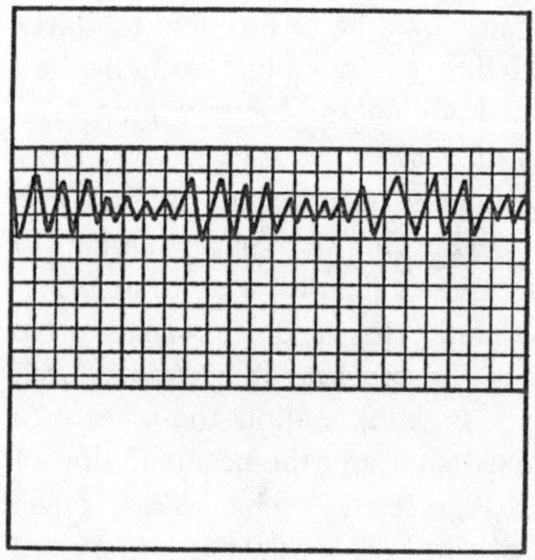

EEG: Normal tracing for a nonsmoker.

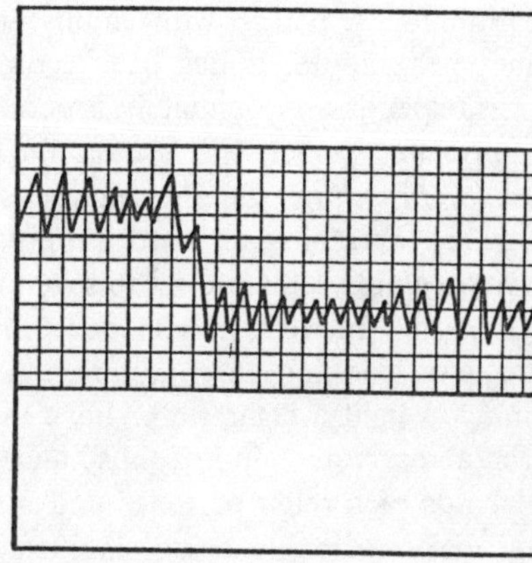

Smoker's EEG: Evidence of reduction in the electrical output of the brain.

This reduction in brain activity is one of the numerous items you can use in your visualization program. Brain function is altered when you smoke. One way to develop a mental image of this is to picture the before and after EEG of a typical smoker.

Skin Wrinkling

At our Wellness Seminars, I usually get the attention of women smokers more quickly on this subject than any other. All of us are vain to some degree. We always want to look as young as possible. If anyone tells you otherwise, you have reason for suspicion. This is one of the reasons interest is high when considering the role of smoking in skin wrinkling. Another reason is because it is one of the few harmful effects of smoking which you can *see*.

Why and *how* does smoking cause skin wrinkling? As has been indicated, smoking causes a marked increase in the secretion of epinephrine (adrenaline). Epinephrine is a potent vasoconstrictor which causes the blood vessels to contract. This produces a reduction of blood flow to the skin. This reduction in blood flow reduces the amount of oxygen delivered to the skin. Optimal amounts of oxygen are required for normal function and reproduction of skin cells. When the oxygen is reduced, as it is for smokers, the skin ages faster. This smoking-induced, premature skin aging occurs all over the body but is more pronounced where the skin is exposed to sunlight. Thus "smoker's skin" is most prevalent on the face, neck, hands, and arms. This reduction of oxygen to the skin is another reason why smokers usually have a gray sallow complexion and many cannot blush. So, if you are interested in a face full of premature, deep wrinkling, smoking is the most efficient way to develop it.

I spend a tremendous amount of time in airports. One of my pastimes is observing the facial wrinkling patterns of both men and women. In men, I look at the back of the neck. With women, the sagging skin under the chin. If I notice these two are exaggerated, nineteen times out of twenty the person will either be smoking or will light up within five minutes. Not very scientific, but a subjective observation that smoking causes cosmetic havoc to the face.

In your program of visualization, remember to develop your mind pictures of yourself with and without extensive premature facial skin wrinkling. This is one of the few devastating effects of smoking you can see every time you look in the mirror. Smoking turns your cosmetic clock too fast forward.

Osteoporosis

In addition to speeding up the process of skin aging (wrinkling), smoking can accelerate other conditions usually associated with aging. For example, smokers have been reported to be more prone to develop osteoporosis. Osteoporosis is a bone condition caused by calcium depletion. Though this is a part of the natural aging process, smoking seems to speed it up. With a subnormal amount of calcium, the bones become brittle and break more easily. This condition also causes a general deterioration of the skeletal system and can result in kyphosis, which is a curving of the upper portion of the spine. It is seen fairly often in senior citizens, and in women more often than men. Some think that osteoporosis is more prevalent in women because it may be related to diminished amounts of estrogen after menopause.

There is probably little that can be done to slow down the natural course of osteoporosis, but the main point is that since smoking causes an unnatural depletion of calcium from the bone, the onset of osteoporosis may be speeded up. So, if you think that having a premature stooped shouldered posture is attractive and desirable, smoking may hasten the process. On the other hand, if you want to be sure of straight and erect posture and have healthy bones, stop smoking.

Try to develop this picture in your mind. Smoking acts like a magnet. It draws calcium out of the bone. When this occurs, the aging process of the bone speeds up. Develop the ability to visually picture the calcium in your bones being depleted. Picture your bones becoming fragile. Picture what

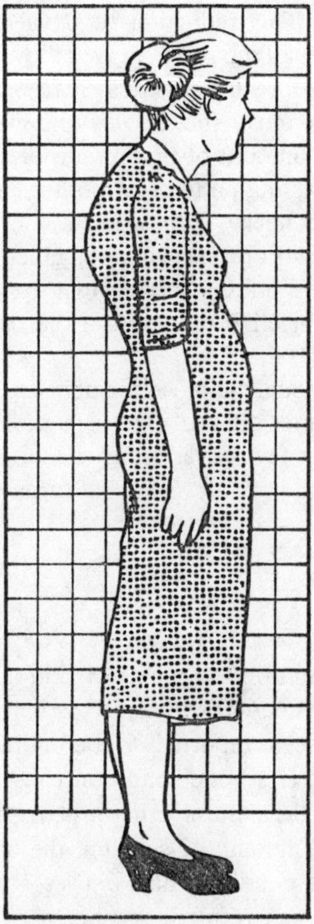

Osteoporosis

you will look like in the future with back and shoulders hunched over due to premature calcium depletion and osteoporosis. Then picture yourself with a strong back and shoulders erect and agile. Get a good clear picture of yourself that way. Do you like it? Do you really want another cigarette?

Vitamin C

Calcium is not the only item which is depleted from the body by smoking. Smoking will rob you of vitamin C. In a two-year study reported by Dr. O. Pelletier including 4,600 men and women, it was found that vitamin C blood levels were 40 percent lower in smokers than in nonsmokers. In the United States, 50 million people may be causing vitamin C deficiency by smoking. There is a vitamin C tax on every pack of cigarettes sold!

Vitamin C is a water-soluble vitamin, which means it is not stored in the body. It takes approximately seventy-two hours for all vitamin C in the body to be used. Add to this the insult of smoking-induced depletion.

Why is this important? Vitamin C is essential for a variety of normal body functions. We need adequate levels of vitamin C in order for iron to be properly used in the transportation of oxygen by the blood. It is essential for good maintenance of bone and muscle tissue. Vitamin C is required for the healing of wounds and fractures. It is necessary for healthy gums and important in our resistance to infection. You must develop the ability to visualize each cigarette flushing necessary vitamin C from your system.

The Unborn Child

Much has been written and said about the effects of smoking on the unborn child. A somewhat paradoxical situation exists between the effect of smoking on the mother and on the unborn child. As has been pointed out, when you smoke you have the accelerator to the floor as you drive the automobile of the aging process. Your skin wrinkles faster, osteoporosis develops quicker, lung problems intensify. The race of aging is finished sooner. Just the opposite seems to occur to the unborn baby. The mother who smokes slams on the brakes of prenatal development. This presents a potentially hazardous situation for the baby. Babies born to smoking mothers are more often born prematurely. A premature baby has less chance for survival. Often, premature babies are kept in the hospital for considerable periods of time. This is worrisome and expensive. When the mother smokes, the baby will be smaller at birth. In addition, a higher incidence of *death in utero* (the baby dying before birth) has been found with mothers who smoke during pregnancy.

Numerous explanations have been brought forth as to how and why a mother who smokes retards the development of her baby and increases the possibility of death before birth. The most logical is involved with oxygen reduction in the blood. The development and growth of a baby in the uterus is indeed one of life's most sophisticated and spectacular marvels. Cellular growth and reproduction is very dependent on oxygen. Oxygen is the magic elixir which is responsible for fetal growth. The only way the unborn baby receives this elixir of life for development and growth is through the mother's blood.

It has already been pointed out how and why smoking reduces the amount of oxygen in the blood. This means less oxygen for the baby. Why is it that mothers who want to provide the very best for their baby continue to smoke? The reason is simple. Most are unaware of the devastating effects on the unborn child.

We know you would do nothing to limit the amount of life-giving oxygen for your baby after it's born; you want it to have every opportunity to grow and mature. But did you know you were unintentionally aiding controlled suffocation for your yet-to-be-born child?

Ambient Smoke

A question which comes up often is about the effect that atmospheric tobacco smoke has on other people. When a nonsmoker (or smoker) is exposed to a room full of tobacco smoke, what *is* the effect?

So-called ambient smoke must be considered in two categories. One is smoke that comes from a burning cigarette—the cigarette placed in an ashtray and allowed to burn. This is the most harmful form of ambient smoke because it has not had the benefit of being filtered through the cigarette itself. This cigarette smoke contains 100 percent of all the harmful ingredients found in burning tobacco. How often have you been in a smoke-filled room and five, ten, or more cigarettes were burning away? This is the most dangerous type of smoke for you, the smoker, and for all the others around you.

The other type of ambient smoke is that which has been inhaled and then exhaled by a smoker. This smoke is almost as harmful to the innocent nonsmoker as to the smoker, the main difference being that the temperature of the exhaled smoke is lower than when taken into the lungs of the smoker. Have you ever stopped to think how hot tobacco smoke is when it enters your lungs? The kindling temperature of cigarette paper and tobacco, which is the temperature required to burn the paper and tobacco, is approximately 380° F. The smoke immediately given off from burning tobacco is that hot. When you inhale a cigarette, the smoke from the burning paper and tobacco is deep in the recesses of your lungs within a fraction of a second. Filtering the smoke through the tobacco in the cigarette cools it some, but your lungs absorb most of this unnatural heat.

Recently a study from Harvard University tested the lung function of children where neither parent smoked, one parent smoked, and both parents smoked. The children, aged five to nine, were given a standard pulmonary vital capacity test. Where neither parent smoked, the children's lungs were normal. Where one parent smoked, there was marked reduction in lung vital capacity, which is a measurement of the amount of air that can be inhaled and exhaled. When both parents smoked, there was significant reduction in the lung vital capacity.

The evidence is strong that ambient smoke is harmful to others around you. You may take a "so what, that's their problem" attitude. If so, and you have children, at least think of them. You may be damaging their lungs for the future.

Speaking of children, another study was published recently from the Harrisburg-Scranton area of Pennsylvania. It pointed out that children of parents who smoke are much more interested in starting the habit themselves than children of nonsmokers. In the study, it indicated that slightly over 25 percent of the children of smokers had started smoking by the age of eight.

WHY DO YOU SMOKE?

Did you ever ask yourself why you smoke? Do you ever wonder what makes you want to light up? I have asked these questions of hundreds of people. A few are honest enough to say, "I don't know." Many indicate, "It gives me something to do with my hands." Some suggest that "Smoking helps me control my appetite." Many simply say, "It's a habit." A small number report that "Smoking helps calm my nerves."

Smokers, like most who have negative lifestyles, can offer dozens of reasons to justify their bad health habit. This is not intended to be critical but to point out that it's human nature to defend a negative lifestyle that is not understood and that seems to provide such pleasure.

The first step you must take before you can stop smoking is to know the real reason you continue to smoke—the real reason you get the urge to light up. *You continue to smoke because you are addicted to nicotine.* Periodic urges to smoke are related directly to the nicotine level in your blood. When the nicotine level in your blood falls below your personal threshold level to satisfy your body needs, it is sensed by the mind. This is another of the body's checks and balances. The mind detects the lowering level of nicotine in the body and sends out the message, "Light up and give me another dose of nicotine." You have no choice. The body cannot think; it always acts in response to the direction of the mind. You will obey your mind signals. After you have taken a few deep inhalations, the nicotine level of the blood rises rapidly. You are giving your body what it's craving—another dose of nicotine! After the nicotine rises above your personal threshold level, the urge or craving is gone. Your body will be satisfied for a certain period of time. Your smoking habit is based upon this roller-coaster ride of nicotine.

That fellow in the old cigarette slogan who would walk a mile for a particular brand wasn't out for the exercise! He needed a nicotine fix and would walk a mile, five miles, ten miles, any distance to have his nicotine level replenished.

The way to break your dependency on nicotine is to educate your mind about exactly how and why smoking is affecting you. Until the present time, your appetite for smoking had no opposition. There was nothing to bring it under control. You can assume that control by learning *how* and *why* smoking is destroying your vital organs and body systems. Remember, until you studied this chapter, the regulators of your body were set for the acceptance of smoking as an okay activity. The body cannot readjust the regulators. Only the mind can accomplish this. Before regulator changes will occur, the mind must be informed, educated, and, indeed, indoctrinated about the relationship between smoking and premature death.

While there may be minor variations in the way smokers respond to the Plan for the Elimination of Negative Lifestyles, the basic reaction is predictable. You will notice at first the urge to light up will be less frequent. This will be a totally unconscious reaction. You will not be thinking about it or trying to space out the time between cigarettes. It just happens. Next, you will find the pleasurable taste of a cigarette will vanish. It will go from your previous "cigarettes taste good" to a neutral sensation. You will find that you experience neither a favorable nor an unpleasant taste sensation. As you find the number of cigarettes you smoke each day declining and the taste response becoming neutral, the most dramatic change starts. *Cigarettes may start to make you slightly nauseated!*

The main point is that the Plan for Elimination of Negative Lifestyles produces a situation in which, through visualization, the mind is finally giving the orders to your body. Once this occurs, everything becomes automatic. Beyond this point, it's out of your hands. Signals are sent out altering your nicotine requirements. Your taste reactions change. Everything is readjusted so that smoking is no longer acceptable. When this occurs, smoking is rejected and you are among the tens of thousands who call themselves ex-smokers.

This system for elimination of smoking may result in a "cold turkey" stop-all-at-once situation. This is the usual way. However, it is important for you to understand that a gradual reduction method is used by many. You must select your own method. Both are equally effective.

As we have collected data, we can predict with a fair amount of accuracy the typical pattern of reduction. It seems as if the first cigarette to be eliminated is the one before breakfast. The last (most difficult) is the one after breakfast.

One of the attractive facets of this Plan is that it is permanent. As long as the visualization program can be recalled so as to reinforce the no smoking signals being sent out, the urge to smoke will not return. Conversely, if you attempt the visualization program without sufficient education and effort, the results will be unsatisfactory in the short and long run. There are no shortcuts for your visualization program. It takes effort, but your smoking days will be over forever.

HOW TO STOP SMOKING

With this as background, we are ready to review, in depth, your Plan for the Elimination of Your Negative Lifestyle—in this case, smoking. As was pointed out in the beginning of this chapter, this program is only for those who truly want to stop smoking. It works every time and once started is out of your control. Your subconscious mind becomes the Maestro who orchestrates your personal symphony to become an ex-smoker.

Step One: *Make your personal commitment to stop smoking.* By now you have already established your list of priorities for the elimination of your negative lifestyles. To stop smoking is number one on your list. You must now make your own personal commitment. It is essential after you have thought through your personal commitment that you write it down.

I have reviewed many of these written commitments. Often I see something like this: "I am totally dedicated to stop smoking. It is one of the most important things in my life. By eliminating this bad health habit from my life, I expect to feel better and live longer." Your written commitment can be as short or as long as you like. The most important thing is for your personal commitment to be the result of your own thought process. It should be in your own words and you should really believe in the commitment.

Remember that your total concentration and commitment must be devoted to stop smoking. I repeat this point because one of the mistakes made most often by those seeking high-level wellness is to eliminate more than one negative lifestyle at the same time. This is a recipe for certain disaster. When it comes to the readjustment of the body's regulators to reject negative lifestyles, the mind works best as a single channel instrument. For this reason, forget for now all other negative lifestyles. Don't allow this restriction to detract from your excitement or enthusiasm but do recognize that you will be working on the elimination of your second negative lifestyle sooner than you think.

Step Two: *Study and review again all the material and data in this chapter.* This is one of the most important of all steps for the elimination of your smoking habit. I want you to go back and reread and study all the material presented in this chapter. I want you to have a clear *understanding* of every single effect that smoking has on destroying your vital organs and inhibiting your body systems. Learn the proved statistics about the increase in lung cancer. Study and understand all actions of nicotine on the body—what it does and why.

Become an expert on the action of carbon monoxide—what it does to the blood and the effect on each organ. Learn in detail the relationship between smoking and cardiovascular diseases, bronchopulmonary diseases, premature skin wrinkling, and osteoporosis. Know about the effect of smoking on the unborn and how and why ambient smoke is harmful. This is the opportunity of a lifetime! A nice, neat package with all the information you need.

Step Three: *Develop the ability to mentally* visualize *cigarette smoke destroying your vital organs and body systems.* You are provided with numerous illustrations in this chapter. The purpose of these artists' concept drawings is to give you a simple mental interpretation of what happens to your vital organs and body systems when you smoke. You are always provided with a companion illustration which shows what the same vital organs or body systems look like in a nonsmoker. In other words, one illustrates for you the disease or unhealthy state induced by smoking and the other the healthy disease-free condition of the nonsmoker.

Now that you understand all the information about how smoking affects your body, go back and study the illustrations carefully. I want you to be able to mentally recall what the normal, healthy state for your various vital organs and body systems looks like. Be able to develop a vivid mental picture of each and every minute detail. Next, do the same for the illustrations depicting the vital organs and body systems of the smoker. This is what's going on inside your body! Give particular attention to the differences between normal and unhealthy.

Here is the key to this program. You must be able to mentally visualize what your hemoglobin looks like as it is deprived of oxygen by your smoking-induced carbon monoxide loading. Get a mental picture of your adrenal glands pouring forth epinephrine as the nicotine builds in the blood—of the responses to this—contraction of the blood vessels—heart racing faster—blood pressure going up. Picture on your mental television what happens when your platelets clump together. Picture yourself full of premature facial wrinkles—caused by smoking. You must study and memorize each of the illustrations until you can call forth on command your own personalized mental kaleidoscope of physical changes caused by smoking.

It is the information you provide to the mind and your ability to mentally recall the devastating bodily effects of smoking that motivates your mind to send new signals to the body. These are the signals which will readjust your regulators so that smoking is no longer acceptable.

Step Four: *Write a summary of everything you learn about how and why smoking destroys your vital organs and body systems.* Before starting your visualization program, write a summary of everything you have learned about how and why smoking is harmful. The learning process is faster and retained better if more than one of the senses are used. Thus, by reading, mentally condensing, and writing a summary, the mind is more quickly informed and indoctrinated as to why you should stop smoking.

If you like, do the same thing with the illustrations. Many people like to improvise. They use the illustrations in this chapter as a guideline; then they make their own personalized sketches as to how *they* think smoking affects body systems. This is great! The more *you* become involved in creating your own visualization program, the more effective it will be for you. Anatomical correctness is not as important as being able to visualize drastic changes taking place and understanding why the changes occur.

Step Five: *Practice visualization programs every morning upon awaking, noon, evening, just before going to sleep, and every time there is an urge to light up.* Once you have sufficient information and knowledge about smoking to be able to visualize, you must organize your program as to *when* to visualize. Basically, this is an exercise in discipline. The more often you visualize, the more rapidly you will achieve your goal of becoming an ex-smoker.

You should begin by visualizing as soon as you wake in the morning. Condition yourself that before you allow your thought process to start on the matters of the day, do your visualization programs. You will find that within a few days this will come automatically. As soon as your eyes open, you will think of your visualization program. Lie there and think. Visualize everything you know about the harmful effects of smoking. By visualizing first thing in the morning, your day is set. Your mind is saturated and immersed in the water of visualization. Subconsciously you have started a day of instruction for your mind, a day of instruction as to why and how smoking destroys vital organs and body systems.

In regard to the other times of day for visualization, I suggest you tie it in with other routine habits. If you work where there is a morning and an afternoon break, this is an ideal time. Under these conditions, practice visualization before the morning break, before lunch, and before the afternoon break. This system is good because it gives you a definite time each day to tune into your mental drama of how to stop smoking. For most, these breaks in the work day are times for smoking. You will quickly see how your appetite for smoking at these habitual times changes. Notice how the desire for the cigarette with your coffee diminishes.

After you get home, the best time for visualization is before the evening meal and just before going to sleep. The last visualization of the day is probably the most important because the brain continues to function while you sleep. Feed your mind the vitamins of visualization and the signals sent to your body to stop smoking will be strong and healthy.

Don't be surprised if you visualize unconsciously. Most people do. You will find that your visualization program will flash across your mind at unscheduled times. This is great! The more you become involved with visualization, the sooner you will become an ex-smoker.

All of the visualization advice I have given thus far is designed to be used while you are still smoking. Until you have stopped smoking, your visualization program should concentrate only on the harmful effects of smoking—how and why smoking destroys vital organs and body systems.

After you have stopped smoking, there is a change in the program. After your first day of no cigarettes your visualization program should be shifted from pictures of what your vital organs and body systems look like being destroyed by smoking, to what your vital organs and body systems look like in the healthy condition of an ex-smoker. I realize everything does not revert back to normal immediately; however, you should visualize it as if it has. In essence, your new visualization program is what your body will become now that you are out from under the influence of smoking.

Even after you have had a full day without a cigarette, your problems are not over. You will have numerous strong urges to smoke. When this occurs, you should again visualize. Get the picture of your normal healthy state and contrast it with visual pictures of what used to occur to your vital organs and body systems when you were a smoker.

Your schedule for visualization is an important part of the Plan for Elimination of Negative Lifestyles. Practice your newfound skill regularly and diligently and you will be amazed how quickly you become an ex-smoker.

Step Six: *Determine and write down a schedule or target date whereby smoking will be eliminated.* You must have a definite schedule whereby you will stop smoking. This schedule must not be established until *after* you are completely prepared to start your in-depth visualization program. To attempt to establish your countdown to becoming an ex-smoker after scanning the material in this book is a mistake.

In essence, your schedule is your defined goal. Generally speaking, nothing in life is accomplished without a definite goal. To stop smoking is no exception. The signals to readjust your body regulators against smoking will be sent according to the schedule you have established and transmitted to the mind. This is why it is absolutely essential that a schedule for withdrawal be established. If you do not discipline the brain with a definite schedule, the signals will be sent in an undisciplined way.

The first question that presents itself is: What timetable should you establish? This is up to each individual. Some want to go "cold turkey." You can set that date. Others prefer a scheduled reduction. You may want to count the number of cigarettes you smoke tomorrow. After you start the visualization program, your goal may be to reduce the number of cigarettes per day by two or three or four or some other number. I find that those who are confident and self-assured usually go the cold turkey route. Others who are more methodical and achievement-oriented prefer the reduction way. Regardless, both methods work. The main point is for you to establish your goal in a manner that is most comfortable for you.

Step Seven: *Develop a vivid mental image of you not smoking.* Develop the ability to visualize yourself without a cigarette in your hand or mouth, without the panicked feeling of being out without another supply available. Imagine your pockets or purse not bulging with a pack. Think of what it will be like not wondering if you are offending others when you smoke. How about the embarrassment of a long ash and no ashtrays in sight? Think about what it will be like without tobacco taste and smell on your breath. (A friend of mine once said, "Kissing a person who smokes is like tasting a dirty ashtray.") Think about the extra money you will have for other, nonharmful pleasures. Most of all, think of how much better you will feel—your newfound energy. Think about your extra years of life.

By visualizing yourself not smoking, you are giving specific instructions to the mind as to what you want done, what you want to accomplish. With this specific input, you can program your body in a more efficient way that smoking is no longer acceptable as a lifestyle. The mind has a final goal to shoot for: you as you visualize yourself not smoking.

This system works every time provided you are serious and apply each of the steps exactly as described. You may wonder how I can be so sure. It's simple. If you educate and indoctrinate the mind with the information contained in this chapter, establish a schedule, get a picture of yourself not smoking and visualize on a regular basis, the mind will do the rest.

You have no conscious control. Your subconscious mind will be in the driver's seat. It will direct your body to no longer crave nicotine and to reject smoking as a lifestyle.

GOOD NEWS FOR SMOKERS

I have found that after a person has reviewed and become familiar with the Plan to Stop Smoking, a number of questions will be asked. By far the most prevalent is: "How much damage have I already done to my body?" Others want to know: "Can I undo the harm that has already been done?"

The answer for smokers is—good news!—numerous medical studies have pointed out that many of the problems caused by smoking can be almost completely reversed. There are many factors that determine the response you will have as you become an ex-smoker. Some of these factors are your age when you started, the number of cigarettes you have smoked per day, how short you smoke each cigarette, and how long you have smoked.

Regardless, your return to normal health is dependent upon the amount of time which passes without becoming ill. Put another way, the longer you live after you stop smoking, the longer you are going to live. It has been pointed out that cessation of cigarette smoking definitely reduces your risk from cardiovascular diseases and after ten years off cigarettes, your risk approaches that of the person who has never smoked. There is a similar decrease in the risk of lung cancer. After you have been off cigarettes for ten to twelve years, your risk of dying of lung cancer is only slightly higher than for someone who has never smoked. What this data suggests is that you now have available a program which allows you to reverse almost completely all the harm done to your vital organs and body systems. The process of reversal does not occur overnight. It takes time—in fact, years. For this reason, don't let another month or year go by.

Remember what was said about smoking and premature death. Consider those two men aged fifty-five—one who has smoked one or more packs per day for the last thirty years compared with another who has never smoked. The smoker will die eight years sooner. Need anything more be said? Smoking takes years off your life and completely destroys any chance for a high-quality life. By now you know how and why this occurs. Use your newfound knowledge wisely.

About the only good thing to be said for smoking is that, under certain conditions, all or a portion of the harm done to the body can be completely reversed. The way to accomplish this seeming miracle is to start today on your program to eliminate smoking. Regardless of how many times you have tried and failed, you are about to try for the last time. You are about to become an ex-smoker.

YES, YOU CAN STOP SMOKING!

ADDITIONAL HELPFUL HINTS

At the end of each chapter you are provided with a brief outline of practical information, tips, and hints that are intended to supplement your visualization program. When used in conjunction with visualization, it will help you eliminate your negative lifestyle.

These practical tips consist of a number of suggestions and ideas that can help you break the smoking habit.

1) Make it difficult to smoke. Get rid of all your ashtrays. Throw away your lighters and matches.
2) To satisfy oral cravings, keep a container of fresh, raw carrots, cauliflower, radishes, and cabbage in the refrigerator. When away from home use sugarless gum. When you have the urge to light up, take a long drink of cold water.
3) When traveling always sit in the nonsmoking section of the plane, train, or bus.
4) Always refuse any cigarette offered by another person.
5) Newer research points out that the more acidic your body's chemical balance, the faster you flush nicotine out of your system. The faster the smoker loses his nicotine, the more often he wants to smoke. You can reverse this by eating foods which are alkaline (opposite of acid). Foods which are highly alkaline are raisins, dried figs, lima beans, spinach, carrots, lettuce, grapefruit, bananas, oranges, and peaches. In summary, vegetables and fruits are the best body alkalizers, meats are the worst. Stress also increases body acidity.
6) Buy only one pack at a time.
7) Never smoke while in bed, while driving, or while standing.
8) Don't keep a cigarette in your hand. Put it in the ashtray after each puff.
9) Never smoke your first cigarette until after breakfast.
10) Never smoke a cigarette more than half its length.

11) When smoking, concentrate fully on the act of smoking and what it's doing to your body. Don't smoke when you are preoccupied by watching television, working, drinking, or reading.

12) Decide to do one of the following: never smoke alone *or* never smoke in the presence of others.

13) Inhale only every other puff.

14) For one month put aside an amount of money equal to that spent for cigarettes. Realize how much you can save in one year.

15) Establish a reward system for yourself. After you have been off cigarettes for three months, buy yourself a new piece of clothing you have wanted. After six months, something a little more valuable. After one year, plan a long weekend away with someone special.

5 COPING WITH EVERYDAY STRESS

"When I don't have anything to worry about,
I begin to worry about that."
WALTER KELLY

What is stress?

In my travels around the country, I have asked many people this question. Often I get answers like this: "Stress is being told your airplane is two hours late or canceled when you have an important connection on the other end." "Stress is being unemployed with all the monthly bills two weeks overdue." "Stress is having half the test questions on the final exam taken from the last two chapters of the textbook, which I did not study." "Stress is the unexpected death of a close friend or relative." "Stress is being in the middle of a traffic jam when I am already fifteen minutes late for an important meeting." "Stress is anticipating the boss's reaction to the last report I submitted."

What does stress mean to you? Most people cannot precisely define what stress is, though they know that it causes them to feel differently than usual.

While William James did not use the word stress, he may have been describing the end result when he said,

> "Everyone is familiar with the phenomenon of feeling more or less half alive on different days. Everyone knows on any given day that there are energies in him which the incitements of that day do not call forth. Compared with what we ought to be we are only half awake. Our fires are damped, our drafts are checked. We are making use of only a small part of our possible mental and physical resources."

Stress *does* cause you to feel differently. It can drain you of energy. It can cause you to develop and maintain a dark outlook on life. It can destroy your enthusiasm for any activity. It can create an attitude of chronic pessimism deep within your soul.

How great is the problem of stress? Some people recognize anxiety as the result of stress and seek professional help. The National Institute of Drug Abuse estimates that every year 120 million prescriptions are written for tranquilizer drugs. It is estimated this represents 4 billion individual doses per year. The Commerce Department points out that the annual expenditure for tranquilizer drugs accounts for *25 percent of the nation's total drug bill.*

There is a time and a place for tranquilizers and other drugs in treating the symptoms of stress. However, they usually do little to correct the basic problem. To eliminate the cause of the stress, what you need is information and knowledge. Remember, one of the prerequisites for developing wellness self-responsibility is for you to have adequate information, which you can convert into knowledge. You need to know what stress is and how it affects you. You must know *how* and *why* stress affects your vital organs and body systems. You need to know, when subjected to stress, how and why your blood pressure goes up. How and why your heart beats faster and breathing increases. How and why you start to perspire. How and why your face turns red and your stomach starts to rumble.

You need to know what's happening inside your body each time your emotions get out of control. At the present time your body regulators are set to respond automatically to stressful situations. Your program to short-circuit this automatic, body-harming reaction begins with education.

That brings us back to our original question: What is stress?

Dr. Hans Selye, the recognized pioneer in the study of stress, has defined it as "the body's nonspecific response to any demand made upon it." He continues: "Stress is the everyday wear and tear on the mind and body."

I would like to add my definition. *Stress is any internal or external change which has an impact on our sensory perceptions.* The key words are *change* and *sensory*. First, sensory refers to any of our basic senses such as sight, smell, touch, hearing, taste, and emotion. Any condition which causes a noticeable shift or change in the routine to which these senses have become accustomed is stress.

Let's consider specific examples:

Sight

If you have worked a job which takes place in a highly lighted environment and then become an usher in a theater, you encounter a stressful situation. The opposite is also true. If you go from being a waiter in a dimly lit restaurant to working at the city desk of a busy newspaper, you will experience stress.

Smell

If you have worked in the North Woods where the air is fresh and clean and suddenly become chief chicken plucker in a poultry processing plant, stress will become a part of your life. If you have worked at a film-processing company where the odor of certain chemical agents is apparent and then you become a deckhand on an oceangoing vessel where the salt air is always fresh, you will notice stress.

Touch

If you are accustomed to wearing an open-collared shirt or blouse and suddenly switch to a tight or high-collared garment, stress will take its toll. Changing from light summerweight to heavy and coarse winterweight clothing can be a cause of stress.

Hearing

If you work all day in a library and come home to the stereo pouring out 80 watts of hard rock music, you will be stressed to the point of pulling the plug. Have you ever heard the expression that "the silence is deafening"? If you are accustomed to high-level noise and are suddenly subjected to extended periods of silence, the stress is real.

Taste

If you are accustomed to a diet which is basically bland and salt-free and suddenly switch to a diet which is high in salt and spice, you will experience not only physical distress, but also equal amounts of mental stress. If you develop hypertension and your diet has been high in salt, your physician may put you on a low-sodium diet. This reduction in accustomed salt intake can cause stress.

Emotion

Some people will debate if emotion should be considered along with the five basic senses. They point out that emotion is an end product. This is true, but I also contend that your emotion is a receptor, that is, it reacts to changes and therefore should be considered along with the senses when trying to describe the definition. If you suddenly lose a loved one due to death, the stress is obvious and sometimes almost unbearable. When you gain a new loved one due to birth or marriage, the stress is very real.

At the beginning of this chapter, I listed several examples of stress. Stop for a moment. Get a piece of paper and a pencil. Write down as many examples of stress as you can think of.

What do you have on your list? Look at it carefully. Do your examples of stress have anything in common? Are they all negative or unpleasant?

Probably so. This is one of the most elementary mistakes people make. They are of the opinion that stress is always due to something bad.

Happy events can be just as stressful as unhappy events. How about when you get the big promotion you have been after for five years? How about getting married? How about going on that long-awaited four-week vacation? How about buying that new house you have dreamed about so long? Would you relate these occurrences to stress? At first most people say no, but allow me to assure you that stress—and the body's reactions caused by these happenings—is real.

The main point is that *stress is always tied to an event. The event can be pleasant or unpleasant.* Regardless of whether it's pleasant or unpleasant, the event always reflects *change.*

Dr. T. H. Holmes has published the Social Readjustment Rating Scale. In developing the Scale, hundreds of men and women were interviewed and completed questionnaires in which they were asked to rank forty-three life stress events (pleasant and unpleasant). Marriage was assigned an arbitrary point value of 50. With this as a guide, each participant rated the life stress events according to the degree of readjustment required. The following chart is the result:

LIFE EVENTS	SCALE OF IMPACT	LIFE EVENTS	SCALE OF IMPACT
Death of spouse	100	Change in number of arguments with spouse	35
Divorce	73	Mortgage over $10,000	31
Marital separation	65	Foreclosure of mortgage or loan	30
Jail term	63	Change in responsibilities at work	29
Death of close family member	63	Son or daughter leaving home	29
Personal injury or illness	53	Trouble with in-laws	29
Marriage	50	Outstanding personal achievement	28
Fired at work	47	Wife begins or stops work	26
Marital reconciliation	45	Begin or end school	26
Retirement	45	Change in living conditions	25
Change in health of family member	44	Revision of personal habits	24
Pregnancy	40	Trouble with boss	23
Sex difficulties	39	Change in work hours or conditions	20
Gain of new family member	39	Change in residence	20
Business readjustment	39	Change in schools	20
Change in financial state	38		
Death of close friend	37		
Change to different line of work	36		

Change in recreation	19	Change in number of family get-togethers	15
Change in church activities	19	Change in eating habits	15
Change in social activities	18	Vacation	13
Mortgage or loan less than $10,000	17	Christmas	12
Change in sleeping habits	16	Minor violations of the law	11

You will notice that life events which are usually considered to be pleasant, such as retirement, pregnancy, addition of a new family member, and job change, rated high and required a great amount of readjustment.

The purpose of this study was to determine if there is a connection between the events contained in the Social Readjustment Rating Scale and illness. The answer is unequivocally yes. It was pointed out that not only does a correlation exist, but as the *number of life events accumulate so does the incidence of illness*. In one study, the total points of an individual's life events were added. If they had a total score of 150–199 life events within twelve months, they had *mild* life crisis. From 200 to 299 reflected *moderate* life crisis and 300 or more *serious* life crisis. Within two years 37 percent of those with mild life crisis became ill, 51 percent of the moderate group, and 79 percent of those with serious life crisis. From this Dr. Holmes concluded that people tend to get sick when clusters of life events take place. It didn't matter whether these changes are pleasant or unpleasant.

In separate studies Dr. Holmes pointed out that the death rate of widows and widowers is ten times greater during the year after the death of the spouse as compared with a similar control group where death of the marriage partner is not a factor. Similarly, divorced persons are twelve times more vulnerable to illness in the first year following divorce than married people of equivalent age.

Someone once said that the only thing absolutely sure about tomorrow is change. We live in a world of change. Every time we turn around, change stares us in the face. So, if change is constant and stress is related to change, how can you avoid stress? You can't! If you are alive and breathing, you are going to be faced with stressful events. Some of you will encounter stress more often than others, but the point is, we are constantly surrounded by stress and always will be. Don't try to delude yourself into thinking you can create a life where there is no stress. It's impossible. Even those who escape to an isolated island in the South Seas cannot become divorced from stressful events. The sooner you understand that stress is eternal and always present, the sooner you will be able to create and enact programs that will allow you to cope with it.

UNDERSTANDING STRESS

One of the basic problems we encounter as we try to determine why we experience stress is contained within the natural makeup of the body. The problem is that, from a physiological point of view, you have the same body as people who lived thousands or millions of years ago. So far as we can tell, there has been no basic change in human body chemistry since the time of recorded history.

Think back to prehistoric society and the cave man and woman. Those people not only had to survive the elements in crude living conditions, but also were at constant war with prehistoric animals which we can appreciate only in museums. The cave man had no sophisticated weapons, only a club and rocks. The possibility existed that the cave man was often faced with other homo sapiens who, for a variety of reasons, had designs on doing him in. Living was a constant struggle for survival.

When compared to us, those people may have had a differently shaped skull and slightly different facial features. The posture may have been more stooped and they probably had more hair on the body, but *internally, the vital organs and body systems were basically the same as today*.

It's easy to understand that these prehistoric citizens encountered constant threats to life and limb. *These situations often required that the individual respond in one of two ways—either run as fast as possible or fight.* The individual being accosted had to make an instant decision—either pick up a club or other suitable weapon and render the opponent (human or animal) inactive, or turn heel in order to place as much space as possible between the two parties. Hence the term "flight or fight."

The way your body reacts to these stressful or frightening situations is another of your systems of checks and balances. The brain can instantly interpret when danger is at hand. However, before the body can react a number of signals must be sent from the brain to the body. There is not enough time for the brain to sort through all the complicated body changes which must take place, then send out the signals required to accomplish them. When faced with a stressful, frightening, or dangerous situation *everything must happen automatically and instantly*.

In order to achieve this seemingly miraculous and instantaneous change in body function and metabolism, your internal regulators send out the signals to change from a nonstressful to a stressful setting. All this occurs without any conscious thought on your part.

What are the end results of the flight or fight reaction? You have probably heard as many stories as I have on the unbelievable feats of strength and courage which humans can perform under these conditions. Perhaps you have been personally involved. Some of the flight or fight stories are about a 150-pound man carrying a 220-pound man down five flights of stairs in a burning building. There have been proved cases of an individual lifting one side of an automobile off an accident victim. During wartime, numerous documented accounts of heroics far beyond human expectations have been noted.

Researchers have worked on the question of what actually happens—what body changes take place during the flight or fight response.

Permit me to get technical for a moment. The brain can instantly detect stress, danger, or frightening stimuli. This triggers the sympathetic (involuntary) nervous system. Increased amounts of epinephrine are produced. Signals from the hypothalamus cause the pituitary gland (sometimes called the master gland) to become active. In response, a number of hormones are released. Adrenocorticotrophic hormone (ACTH) causes the adrenal glands to produce several hormones which cause alterations in the immune system, control of inflammation, and blood sugar. Vasopressin is secreted which contracts the arteries and causes an increase in blood pressure. Thyrotrophic hormone (TTH) causes increased production of thyroxine from the thyroid gland which causes an increase in overall body metabolism.

What does all this mean? One way to look at it is to consider exactly what is required to get the body in condition for flight or fight. First, tremendous amounts of increased energy are required. In order to provide this extra energy, increased amounts of glucose (blood sugar) and oxygen must be made available. This is accomplished through the epinephrine and other hormones which are produced in response to involuntary signals from the brain. Breathing is increased to bring more oxygen into the body. Glycogen is already stored in the liver. This glycogen is converted to glucose and released into the blood. So now we have a situation in which more oxygen is being brought in by faster breathing and a large amount of glucose is being dumped into the circulatory system. The problem now is how to distribute them throughout the body so the cells can produce more energy. Epinephrine is the answer. It causes a marked increase in heart rate. As the heartbeat increases, the blood moves faster and the distribution of glucose and oxygen to the cells improves.

During flight or fight, your vital organs must function to their maximum state of effectiveness. For this reason the brain, heart, kidneys, liver, and other internal organs must have an increased supply of oxygen- and glucose-rich blood. In order to accomplish this, vasopressin causes peripheral vasoconstriction (narrowing of the arteries) in the arms and legs. When this occurs, blood is "shunted" away from the skin, arms, and legs to the brain and viscera or body cavity where the vital organs are located. This allows these organs to function more efficiently. It also explains why many people turn pale (due to decrease in blood at the skin level) when frightened or are in an unexpected stressful situation.

Another major change that takes place during flight or fight is a general body-wide increase in metabolism. All body functions speed up, from digestion to cellular metabolism to excretion. These actions are caused by increased activity of the thyroid gland.

On rare occasions the body's reaction is so extreme that individuals have literally been frightened to death. In these cases, perhaps because of a prior condition, the body simply could not cope with the internal changes. Documented cases exist in which an individual's hair will become gray or white within a very short period of time following an unexpected stress or fright situation. The main point these cases illustrate is that when a person is faced with a frightening or stressful situation, definite and dramatic changes are taking place within the body.

Today we are not faced with the stress of primitive living conditions, enemy warriors, or wild animals. Today our stress can be caused by trying to make financial ends meet, trying to please the boss or wife or friend, making good grades, trying to get that promotion, the unexpected death of your best friend, or trying to lose thirty pounds. Regardless of the stress, the body always reacts the same way. Refer back to the Social Readjustment Rating Scale. Each life stress event listed causes the *same* internal reactions as the cave man experienced with his stress situations. *The main difference is that we cannot physically fight back nor can we run away. We have no release valve.* We have no way to expend the tremendous buildup of tension and frustration caused by the body's reaction to everyday stress.

It's like being in a powerful sports car with one foot on the accelerator pushing it to the floor, while the other foot is on the brake holding all this generated energy stationary. Something has to give.

HOW THE BODY ADJUSTS TO STRESS

Now you know how the flight or fight syndrome gets the body revved up and ready to react to stress. But what happens if you can't respond—can't run or fight? Does the body have a method to determine that you can't and then suddenly shuts down the reaction to stress? In some cases, yes. Although it does not happen suddenly, if you are exposed to a *single* stressful situation, the body can ultimately return to normal. The problem is that we do not live in a society where we are exposed to an occasional stressful event. We are constantly bombarded with many stresses on a daily basis. There is a continual reigniting of the flight or fight process. For this reason, until you can react or take some action to dissipate the generated internal energy, the body remains in a state of frenzy. As the internal reaction to stress converts from an acute reaction to a chronic one, increased blood pressure can become permanent. Those who are borderline diabetics become full-blown diabetics. Duodenal ulcers develop as a result of chronic increased gastric acid production. Resistance to bacterial and viral infection is reduced so that infectious diseases become more of a problem. Since the heart is constantly stimulated to work harder with less oxygen available, the chance of heart attack increases. Because of alterations in the immune system of the body, newer research suggests there might be an increase in cancer. Dr. Selye calls this entire chronic stress process the *exhaustion reaction phase.*

I hope you are beginning to understand the devastating impact that chronic stress can have on your health. From 80 to 85 percent of all mental and physical illnesses are in some way related to chronic stress. High-level wellness will be impossible for you until you learn how to cope with everyday stress.

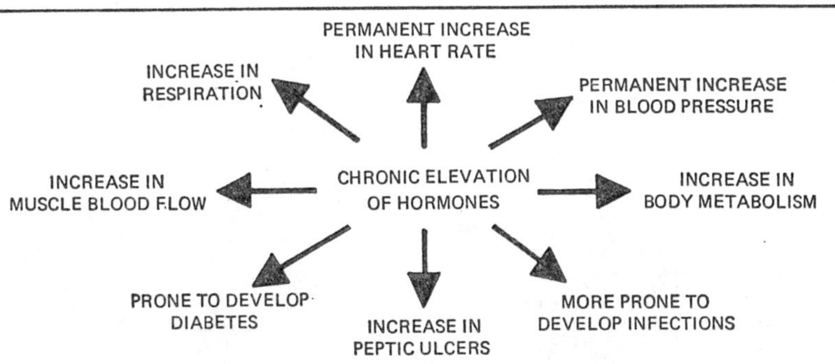

EXHAUSTION REACTION PHASE

Above is an illustration of several of the end results of chronic stress. Become familiar with each of them. Be able to visualize each of them occurring to you.

Reaction to Stress

Have you ever noticed how differently people react to stress? How some people can take it in stride and others become uncontrollably upset or nearly incapacitated? Why do these tremendous variations occur? Let me try to explain.

First, the stressful event itself is not harmful. The event is external. Marcus Aurelius once said, "If you are distressed by anything external, the pain is not due to the thing itself, but to your estimate of it. This you have the power to revoke at any time."

Death of a family member, getting fired, getting married—these events in themselves do not and cannot harm you. It's your reaction to the event that causes trouble. When a stressful event *develops the potential* to become harmful to you personally, it becomes a *stressor*. When the stressor becomes emotionally charged for *you,* when you take it inside, when it becomes a part of you, it is transformed into *distress*. Now you are in trouble because the distress becomes a part of your everyday life. It is the distress that leads to tension, anxiety, and frustration.

Some people have a very low threshold for converting the stressor to distress. Then every stressful event becomes a stressor, and every stressor is converted to distress. These are the people who are tense, anxious, and frustrated all the time. Others have a natural ability to resist this entire process. These fortunate individuals have the ability to maintain life in its proper perspective, and distress seldom is a major problem.

This entire chain of events as first described by Dr. Selye can be illustrated in the following diagram:

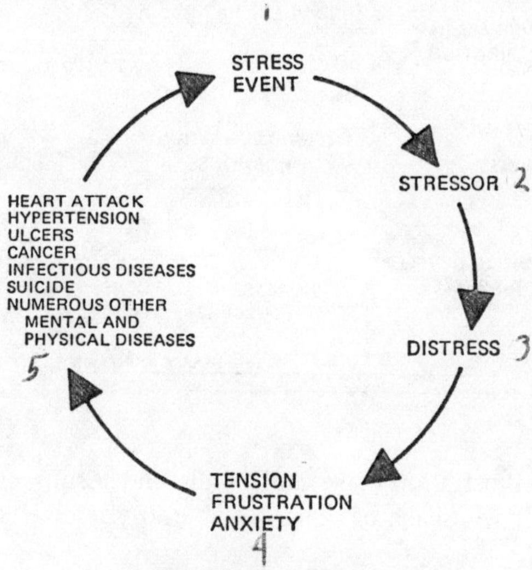

STRESS CYCLE

When the cycle is allowed to mature and continue, the illness or medical problem can become a stressful event unto itself. Now the cycle is never-ending unless a conscious effort is made to break it.

Premature Aging

Another way to think about distress is to realize that its effect on the body causes premature aging. Premature aging is the way you get to premature death.

Of all the negative lifestyles, distress probably speeds up the aging process more than any other. The body was not designed to withstand the constant damage that is caused by the bombs of distress. All of it—abnormal physiological changes and damage caused by distress—simply causes the body, the vital organs, and body systems to wear out sooner. There is not time for sufficient recovery, repair, and maintenance. Every encounter with distress leaves a new scar. The mind and body age prematurely.

HOW TO COPE WITH EVERYDAY STRESS

The problem of dealing with everyday stress is not like the other negative lifestyles addressed in this book. In the case of smoking, excessive consumption of alcohol, obesity, and poor nutrition the goal is to remove something from the lifestyle in order to achieve high-level wellness.

Stress is different. It is impossible to eliminate stress from your lifestyle; nor can you remove yourself from stress. For this reason, high-level wellness is achieved by engaging in a plan that allows you to *cope with* everyday stress so as to minimize its impact on your life. Since the format used for the elimination of other negative lifestyles will not work for stress, we must have a plan designed exclusively for stress.

As you read through the following pages, you will find the **Plan for Coping with Everyday Stress.** The information for the first step has already been provided.

Step One: Learn what stress is, what causes distress, and how and why distress destroys vital organs and body systems.

Step Two: Learn to recognize when you do and do not have control over your worry.

Step Three: Learn how you can conquer the worry over which you do have control and how to put your mind at ease with those you can't control.

Step Four: Become an expert on the role of exercise and meditation in coping with distress.

Step Five: Experiment with techniques for stress control.

Step Six: Establish what your routine for coping with stress will be.

Step Seven: Write down the schedule of when you will be able to cope with stress.

Step Eight: Visualize yourself completely free from the problems of stress.

You have already read and studied the material required for Step One. The information for the remaining steps follows.

To Worry or Not to Worry?

This is the first mention of worry. It is important to consider worry because most people understand the term worry much better than the terms stress and distress. If you don't believe this, ask yourself: How often have I said, "Boy, I am really worried about . . ."? Can you ever remember saying, "Gee, am I stressed (or distressed) over . . ."? The point is that as soon as I say the word worry, you have something familiar to work with.

Is there a difference between distress and worry? Yes. Worry is what causes distress to grow and magnify itself. I define worry as *the excessive preoccupation with a specific relevant or irrelevant issue.* Worry is the catalyst that causes the stressful event (pleasant or unpleasant) to be converted to distress. The stressful event may be a relevant or irrelevant issue. The difference between the two is that you have control over the relevant issues but none over the irrelevant ones. Worry is consciously or unconsciously keeping those issues on the front burner of your thought processes all the time.

Let's consider several examples. If you are two months behind with your automobile payments and worried about it, that's a relevant issue because, ultimately, you have the ability to do something to solve the problem. You can rebudget your money, get a second job, or refinance. On the other hand, if tomorrow is the day of the big annual golf tournament and you are irritated and upset because the weather forecast calls for a 100 percent chance of rain all day, that's an irrelevant issue. Regardless of what you do, nothing is going to change the weather.

See the difference? Worry is so natural and routine that many never take the time to separate the relevant from the irrelevant issues. They never try to separate those issues they have control over from those over which they have no control. You might say that the second step in your Program to Cope with Everyday Stress is to become convinced that there are two different kinds of worries.

From now on you must recognize your controllable worry. This is a worry that responds to action on your part. The other kind of worry is uncontrollable worry. This is excessive preoccupation with an irrelevant issue—one over which you have no control. This worry never involves action—just constant mental agitation, which magnifies the issue 100, 1,000, or 10,000 times.

When separating your controllable and uncontrollable worries, you must learn to ask yourself this simple question: "Is there *anything* I can do to remove this worry from my life or alter it so that it is reduced and has less impact on my life?" If so, it is a controllable worry. If you find the answer is no, you know you have an uncontrollable issue.

Your Worry Card

Starting now, you must learn how to distinguish between worries over which you do and do not have control. In order to do this I want you to carry with you at all times a blank card. If you like, call it a "worry card." At the top of one side write, "Controllable Worries." On the top of the other side write "Uncontrollable Worries." Every time you find yourself preoccupied with a worrisome thought or situation, I want you to thoroughly analyze the situation and determine if this is an issue that is or is not under your control. If it is controllable, enter it on that side of the card with a brief sentence describing the worry and *why* it is controllable. If you determine that you have no control over the worry, do the same on the other side of the card. The most important thing is for you to know and write down *why* it is controllable or uncontrollable.

What is the purpose of this exercise? It's simply a technique that trains you to *discipline* yourself to routinely *analyze* your worries and *recognize* the difference between the controllable and the uncontrollable.

Uncontrollable Worry

For some, just recognizing that a worry is uncontrollable is enough to remove it from the thought process. However, for most, this won't work.

What you must do now is become active in getting your subconscious mind involved in removing the uncontrollable worry from your life. At the present, your mind cannot distinguish between controllable and uncontrollable worry because your mental regulators are set to worry about all (controllable and uncontrollable) distress situations.

The way you readjust your worry regulators is to inform your subconscious mind. The starting point for this is with your "Worry Card." To communicate with your subconscious mind, you must have a quiet time. The best time is at the end of the day, just before going to sleep. Make arrangements so you can be undisturbed and quiet for fifteen to twenty minutes. Review your "Worry Card" for the uncontrollable worries. Think through in detail those worrisome situations and *why* you have no control.

After you are completely convinced that you are correct in your conclusion, tell your subconscious mind something like this: "This is a situation over which I have absolutely no control. My actions or concerns will in no way influence this situation. This worry is removed from my thought process and will no longer be a part of my life." Repeat your statement over several times. Remember, you are giving a command to your subconscious mind.

Next, I want you to visualize yourself without a worry in the world. Picture yourself with a big smile instead of the worried frown. While visualizing, develop the *feeling* of being lighthearted and happy. Visualize yourself with the effervescent *feeling* of being alive and looking forward to tomorrow.

Uncontrollable worry resides in the subconscious mind. Now that you've become aware of it, you will begin to be able to control it. This program helps you to educate and instruct your mind to be unconcerned about uncontrollable worry and through visualization gives it direction toward the result you expect.

Controllable Worry

How do you deal with controllable worry? The answer is *action.* Your greatest enemy in the war against controllable worry is *procrastination.* The way you win the war is to *attack* the worry immediately.

Just as with uncontrollable worry, the answer to solving the problem of controllable worry is to engage the subconscious mind. You must have a quiet time in order to communicate with the subconscious. Your quiet time should be in the evening, just before going to sleep. Review your "Worry Card" for controllable worries. Do an in-depth mental analysis of why you have determined this is a controllable worry. Remember, every controllable worry is nothing more than *a problem for which there is a solution.* During your quiet time, let your mind soar as it seeks solutions to the problem. Then listen to the answers. It may be the next day or next week. Once you employ the subconscious mind to find a solution, it works twenty-four hours a day. However, it still may take time.

After you have found the answer for dealing with your controllable worry, you must act immediately. Start the wheels in motion to remove the controllable from your life and do it without delay.

While you are solving the problem, you must visualize the solution working successfully. Get a mental picture of you going through the actions to achieve the solution. Visualize the problem already solved. Picture in your mind you, as you will be without the controllable worry to bother you. Give your subconscious instructions as to what you want to accomplish.

This entire process of how to remove controllable and uncontrollable worry through quiet time activities and visualization is Step Three in your Plan to Cope with Everyday Stress.

Before proceeding to the next step, I want to present four techniques that will be essential for your overall program. Please understand that these four techniques are in addition to your program to distinguish between controllable and uncontrollable worry. Since you are exposed to many new distresses on a daily basis, you must become involved in additional activities which will protect you from the arrows of distress. This is accomplished by:

- Exercise
- Quieting Techniques
- TM and Mantra
- Visual Imagery

I am not suggesting that all of these will become a part of your program. A certain amount of experimentation on your part must take place so you can determine which of these techniques are best suited for you. I caution you not to try and prejudge the viability of these activities. The only way you can tell if they are to become a part of your program is to determine if they are effective for you.

At the present time, distress controls you. What you must do is perfect your own program that will allow you to break the distress cycle. This won't be easy, but stop and think. A life free from worry, tension, anxiety, and frustration. Isn't that worth expending your efforts on?

Exercise

If I could introduce you to only a single technique for coping with distress, it would be regular sustained exercise. It is probably the least expensive and most effective of all techniques to break the distress cycle. If you become involved in a vigorous exercise such as jogging, swimming, riding a bicycle, or walking, there is no way you can remain tense. Muscles which are exerted must respond with relaxation. If you keep up this exertion-relaxation cycle long enough, the constant tension will be broken.

Exercise works in another way to help overcome your stress. When you are preoccupied with a worrisome situation, your stress builds and builds. The more you think, the bigger it becomes. What you must have is a technique to break your mental concentration cycle. Extended exercise requires concentration. If your exercise program causes you to concentrate on the effort you are expending, you'll find you won't be thinking about your distress. The cycle will be broken. It's really that simple. Extended exercise automatically draws your concentration away from your distress. When finishing a session of regular exercise, you will almost always feel refreshed, elated, and perhaps even slightly euphoric. You will have been successful in cracking the physical and mental tension cycles.

A word of caution about your exercise program. An entire chapter in this book is devoted to physical fitness. It is suggested that you read that chapter before you start any exercise program. If you have been sedentary (not exercised for a period of time) you must go slow! Don't make the mistake of becoming overly enthusiastic about your exercise program and overdo it and hurt yourself. Then you will be worse than before. If you become injured or perhaps aggravate a medical condition, you will wind up with more distress.

I have spoken with people who have tried exercise in order to cope with stress, and they tell me it doesn't work. When I hear this, my first question is always, "How much do you exercise?" Usually I hear, "I jog for five minutes," or "I walk around the block." Some say, "I ride my bike for ten minutes," or "I swim two laps in the pool." It is true that a little exercise may be better than no exercise, but this amount does not provide sufficient exertion to break the distress cycle.

The types of exercise mentioned thus far (jogging, swimming, cycling, walking) are ideal for coping with stress because they are sustained and therefore are not only good in allowing you to adjust to your distress but also excellent for development of cardiopulmonary efficiency. These are not the only good exercises. Some people take particular pleasure in competitive exercise—those involving another person. There seems to be a therapeutic effect in winning. Often these exercises involve the physical act of striking or throwing an object (tennis, racquetball, golf, or hand ball). The actual striking or hitting out allows you to dispense some of your hostilities and frustration. But it must be remembered, the exercise must be sustained so that your concentration is removed from the distress and directed toward the game or activity.

Dr. Paul Dudley White, one of the world's authorities on cardiac medicine and himself a practitioner of daily exercise (riding his bicycle), once stated: "Muscular fatigue, if not excessive, is the best sedative known to man—the best antidote for nervous strain. Sleep is favored and a delicious tranquility results."

There is yet another reason extended exercise allows you to cope with stress. Extended, sustained exercise is the best and most simple technique known to provide a natural channel for the elimination of all the pent-up energy caused by stress. Remember, you have little control over the body's natural reaction to distress. You have become a walking time bomb—just waiting for the right situation to ignite your fuse. Extended, sustained exercise requires extra energy. You have now developed and designed your own release valve. You now have your natural channel for the elimination of your excess energy.

There's another, medical explanation for why sustained exercise works. As you know, the basic cause of the chain of events causing the buildup of energy is the release of large amounts of epinephrine and other hormones into the blood. During extended, sustained exercise, the heart pumps faster. Blood is pushed through the body faster and, on each circuit, passes through the liver and kidneys. Since the liver is the organ of detoxification and the kidneys are the organs of excretion, the hormones are actually cleansed from your body faster. When this occurs, you are getting at the real cause, and that's why exercise is indeed a very effective therapeutic tool.

Other positive effects of exercise in helping you cope with your distress are:

- Your body will become more attractive. Your muscles will firm up and you will lose weight. This will increase your pride, self-esteem, and self-satisfaction.

- Exercise provides you with new goals and objectives. Whether you are a runner, tennis player, bicycle rider, swimmer, walker, or racquetball player, you will soon find that you want to do better. You want to improve. You want to run, walk, bicycle, or swim farther, perhaps faster. These newfound goals and objectives are another mental diversion away from your constant preoccupation with your distress.

- Exercise causes muscular fatigue and promotes sleep. One of the complications of distress is insomnia. You just lie there and, with constant and total concentration, allow the distress to grow and become bigger. With regular exercise, you will sleep better and get the rest you need to tackle your problems while awake.

As I have elaborated in the chapter on physical fitness, the time of exercise is important. I am of the opinion that the best time is after work and before the dinner meal. I know there are many who exercise the first thing in the morning. If you have success with this schedule, stick with it. The reason I prefer the evening is because the frustrations, anxieties, and hostilities of the day are at a maximum level, therefore easier to expel. Second, the muscular tiredness and relaxation is still pronounced at bedtime.

Quieting Techniques

Dozens of books have been written on the plethora of methods for meditation and relaxation. The theory behind meditation is that it provides you with a disciplined method to break the distress-concentration cycle. You can then regain control of your mental processes so that the distress is placed in proper perspective.

Some of the specific methods which have been described are Zen Buddhism, Transcendental Meditation (TM), Yoga, progressive relaxation, and relaxation response. Some experts think hypnosis falls into this same category.

One of the problems with the various forms of meditation is that it is not easy to become proficient. It's one of those activities that sounds easy but requires discipline. We have been trained from childhood that "an idle mind is the devil's workshop." We are told we should constantly be using our brain to think. This is true, but the important thing for you to realize is the difference between disciplined positive thinking and undisciplined, uncontrolled, constant negative thinking. To command the mind to be absolutely blank or to concentrate on a single subject for extended periods of time requires a readjustment on your part. That's the reason many meditation methods require a teacher, either one-to-one or with a group. The teacher serves as a constant source of stimulation for you as you discipline and direct your powers of concentration into new channels.

I am not suggesting that a teacher is required for you to become proficient in methods of meditation. I am suggesting it will require effort on your part to master a technique.

With this background on quieting techniques, let's consider several specific exercises that have been described and used successfully in helping individuals to cope with stress.

TM and Mantra

One approach to transcendental meditation (TM) is to use a mantra. Mantra is a Hindu word. The mantra is used in prayer and incantation. Mantra is a word that is repeated over and over during TM.

The practice of mantra is done as follows. You must be in a quiet place without outside interruption or distractions. You should make yourself as comfortable as possible. Some recommend that you should relax in a comfortable lounge chair. Others say sit upright in a straight-backed chair. You will have to determine which is best for you. The object of mantra is to repeat silently to yourself a word (mantra). You may choose any word that has a pleasant connotation and sound for you. Some research has been done to determine if there are good and bad mantras. Apparently there are. Doctors Furst and Mone, specialists in the practice of TM, have determined that mantras such as om, one, shirm, lum, hum, love, sky, and fly are pleasant and most often used. The only rule is to select a word that is pleasant for you.

The mantra used most often is the word "one." Let's assume this is your mantra. After you are in your selected place and are as relaxed as possible, start to repeat to yourself the word "one." Do it over and over. You should have your eyes closed with full concentration on listening to the word "one." Try and discipline yourself not to allow other thoughts to enter your mind. (This is the difficult part.) With discipline, effort, and training, you will be able to shut out distractions as your ability to focus on your mantra increases. The mantra becomes your vehicle for entering and maintaining your state of relaxation. By developing the ability to devote total concentration to your mantra, you will be diverted from your distress. Thus, you have at your disposal another technique for breaking the concentration-distress cycle.

It is recommended that TM mantra be practiced for a minimum of twenty minutes each morning and evening. You will find that in the beginning your thought process will wander. You will have difficulty in concentrating on the mantra. Don't be discouraged. It takes practice to discipline your mind to remain on a given subject for extended periods. You will find with each TM mantra session that the time you can constantly concentrate on your mantra will increase. Within a reasonable period of time, you will be able to relax and devote twenty minutes or more to mantra-oriented concentration. This will provide you with the break you need to remove yourself from your distress.

Visual Imagery

Visual imagery is similar to TM mantra except that instead of having a word you repeat over and over, you develop a mental picture of a place where you have been—a place where you have actually experienced peace, relaxation, and calm. It might be a mountaintop retreat, a beach, a Caribbean cruise—a place that reflects positive experiences and attitudes.

After you are comfortable in your quiet environment, close your eyes and think back to this place. Develop a detailed mental picture. Devote your entire concentration to your "pleasure place." Again, as you first try this visual imagery, you will find it is difficult or impossible for you to concentrate for extended periods. Your mental replay will be interrupted numerous times with other subjects, which flash across your mind and command your concentration. The more you practice visual imagery, the more proficient you will become in concentrating for protracted periods.

The theory behind this use of visual imagery is similar to the TM mantra. It gives you a disciplined method whereby you divorce yourself from the constant distress-concentration cycle you are in. By practicing visual imagery at least twenty minutes each morning and evening, you regain control of your thoughts and concentration. You have been concentrating constantly on your distress. The more you think about it, the larger it becomes until soon your distress seems to be the largest thing in your life. Visual imagery provides a technique that may put things back into proper perspective. This may be a valuable technique for you as you develop your program to cope with everyday stress.

Planned Response

Stress is an occurrence related to a pleasant or unpleasant event. The stress of some of these events can be anticipated. For example, we know that when a son or daughter gets married, it is a stressful event. A job promotion can be stressful. Giving a speech provides so much stress that some find it almost impossible to do. Knowing that the mortgage payment is coming due with no money in the bank can be a stressful event. I could go on. The point is that even though many stressful events can be anticipated, they are ignored until the last moment—until it is too late to do something about them.

Planned response simply means doing everything possible to get yourself ready so that the stressful event will cause as little distress as possible. When you find yourself taking an examination, giving a speech or presentation before other people, firing someone, being the hostess for a dinner party, be as well prepared as possible. You must study, have all the facts possible, anticipate, plan, project. The better your preparation, the less the chance for distress.

YOUR PERSONAL PLAN FOR COPING WITH STRESS

We are now ready to start your personal program for coping with everyday distress. Your days of excess worry, anxiety, and tension are numbered. You are about to join that select group of people who know how to enjoy life to the fullest.

Step One: *Make your personal commitment to learn how to cope with everyday stress.* You have already examined and analyzed all your negative lifestyles and determined that learning how to cope with everyday stress is at the top of your list. This should be one of the most important objectives of your life.

I want you to think about just how important it is for you to learn to cope with stress. Then write your thoughts down. It isn't important for you to share your written thoughts with anyone else. Just make sure it's sincere and in your own words. It can be several sentences or pages in length. That's not important. The main point is that you make a personal commitment that is a promise to yourself to devote 100 percent of your energies to learning to cope with stress.

Don't be concerned with any of your other negative lifestyles at this time. Put them completely out of your mind. Learning how to cope with everyday stress must have your complete and undivided attention.

Step Two: *Learn what stress is, what causes distress, and how and why distress destroys vital organs and body systems and causes premature aging and death.* The basic reason you have problems with distress is because you don't understand it. The most important single factor in learning how to cope with everyday stress is for you to fill your mind with information about what causes distress. You must become your own expert on knowing and understanding how and why distress destroys vital organs and body systems, how and why distress completely prohibits high-level wellness and contributes to premature aging and death.

Understand and accept the fact that you cannot escape from stress, which surrounds you constantly. Know that the stressful events or stressor in itself is not harmful. It is when the stressor becomes internal and converts to distress that your problem starts. Learn how and why the numerous hormonal and physiological body changes occur. Know how and why these body changes can lead to virtually every physical and mental disease known.

The key to what you must do is to comprehend that the problem of distress is cyclic in nature and that at the present time this cycle has control over you. The secret is for you to understand that this cycle can be broken. Once this occurs, you have started the program that allows you to gain control.

Step Three: *Separate your worries over which you have control from those that are beyond your control.* The greatest problem most people have is not being able to distinguish between controllable and uncontrollable worry. The reason is not because they can't be recognized, but because most people don't understand why they should be divided. What you need is a disciplined program that allows you to analyze and evaluate each of your major worries. Then you can quickly determine if you do or do not have control.

Carry your "Worry Card" with you at all times. Each time you find yourself preoccupied with a relevant or irrelevant issue, think through the situation. You will be amazed how quickly and often you will conclude, "There is really nothing I can do to alter this situation." In many cases you will determine, "Yes, there is a solution to this problem. All I need to do is . . ."

When you make a determination like the former, summarize the entire situation in one sentence as to *why* you have no control and write it on your Worry Card. To this add the following statement: "I am not going to worry about this issue anymore." Do the same for your controllable worries. In one sentence state exactly what you are going to do to solve the problem, and write it on your card.

The fear of worry freezes people into inactivity. Your Worry Card will help you to act on your worry, or to put it out of your mind.

Step Four: *Working with controllable and uncontrollable worries.* At the end of every day, you must review your Worry Card. How many entries do you have? Let's assume you have one of each. You should deal with the uncontrollable one first. Get yourself into a comfortable position, just as if you were going to practice TM. Relax completely and breathe deeply. After your body is relaxed and your mind clear, review in detail your uncontrollable worry. Is it really uncontrollable? If so, you will quickly understand why and become deeply convinced of your lack of control. Then you must instruct your subconscious mind that the issue will never again preoccupy your thinking.

Now you must visualize what your life will be like to be totally free from your uncontrollable worry. Visualize waking up in the morning without this preoccupation. Visualize how different and good you will feel with this extra burden removed.

After you have gone through this exercise to remove uncontrollable worry from your mental processes, you will experience a very relaxed and peaceful sensation. It really is like removing a very heavy weight from your shoulders. At last you have learned how to identify and purge from your lifestyle those worries over which you have no control.

Now you are ready to attack the worry that is listed on your card as being controllable. Again, you must be in a relaxed and meditative posture. In your relaxed mood, think through the situation and review again why you feel it is a controllable worry. Next, consider in detail exactly what the solution is and the exact actions you are going to take.

Visualize the solution as if it has already taken place. Visualize the happy outcome you expect. As you visualize the desired solution, do it within a definite time frame. Is the solution going to take days, weeks, or months? Be sure you provide the subconscious mind with a deadline by which you expect the problem to be solved. *Then you must immediately begin your plan of action.*

Step Five: *Learn about and experiment in order to determine the role of exercise and meditation in coping with stress.* One of the most important questions you must answer is: Where does exercise fit into your program for coping with stress. Exercise is probably the single most effective technique, but only you can determine if it is for you. In order to do this, you must start to become involved in a regular exercise program. After a week or so of exercising, you can determine: Are you feeling better? Are you sleeping better? Do you have more energy? Do things seem to be more in proper perspective?

Based upon the experience of most other people, exercise does all of these things. If you have been sedentary, you must first read chapter 9. Here you will find all of the information needed to safely get you started. The main point is that when you are just starting an exercise program, go slow. Don't try to condition in one week a body that has taken ten years to become deconditioned.

There is only one way to determine which of the quieting techniques is best for you. Experimentation is the answer. As you begin your practice program, it is important for you to realize that becoming proficient in relaxation techniques is not easy. Just as it takes time and effort to convert the body from a deconditioned to a conditioned state, it also takes time and effort to gain control over your mental processes.

Practice the TM-mantra and visualization techniques. They may not be for you, but you will never know until you try. Once you grasp the general idea of the quieting technique, you may want to change or modify the technique. That's fine. The main point is to have a technique that will allow you to break the distress-concentration cycle and regain mental control.

Step Six: *Establish your overall program schedule.* As previously mentioned, your program for review, plan for action, and visualization of controllable and uncontrollable worries should take place on a regular schedule.

By now you have decided if you are going to become involved in an exercise and/or quieting technique program. If so, the biggest mistake you can make is to approach these programs without a schedule. You should exercise at least four times a week. The type and amount of exercise is up to you. The main point is to exercise on a regular schedule until you are pleasantly tired. Your quieting program should be practiced every morning and evening (in conjunction with the worry program). Most recommend that twenty minutes be devoted to each session. I have talked with many who prefer shorter but more frequent sessions. During the day when they feel tension building, they stop, prop their feet on the desk, relax, and practice quieting for five minutes. Try it, you may be amazed how effective this technique is for breaking your mental distress-concentration cycle. It allows you to put things in proper perspective by taking a five-minute vacation away from the distress at hand.

Step Seven: *Determine and write down a time schedule when you will be able to routinely cope with everyday stress.* This may seem like a tall order, one that is impossible. If you have been burdened by distress and worry for many years, how can you possibly establish a date when you can cope with it? Maybe you can't but you must try.

You need a positive, forward-thinking attitude to assist you. You should also try to develop the ability to determine if you are making progress. Do you sleep better? Do you find that your entire thought process is no longer preoccupied with a single worrisome subject? Do you find you can really relax? Do you look forward to and anticipate positive events occurring in your life?

It will not take you long to determine if you are winning the skirmishes and battles in your war against distress. Have a definite written goal for each of the victories and a stated time objective when you can truly cope with your everyday stress.

Step Eight: *Visualize the mental picture of you completely free from the problems of stress.* From the beginning, you must start to mentally visualize yourself as a new more relaxed and carefree person. You now recognize and understand the problems of distress. You know how to work with controllable and uncontrollable worry. Now you must start visualizing you without the symptoms and problems these conditions cause.

You must give your mind a target to shoot at. Give it a picture of you as you want to become. The body always responds to messages from the brain. Your task of readjusting your body's response to distress will be easier if you precondition the mind as to what you expect as an end result—the ability and skill to cope with or adjust to everyday distress.

Soon you will be in a position to establish and perfect your own personal program. This will be accomplished without drugs or outside help. You have within yourself everything required to live a distress-free life. Your no-cost bonus is that you have at your fingertips the answer to prevent premature aging. From now on, you are COPING WITH EVERYDAY STRESS!

ADDITIONAL HELPFUL HINTS

At the end of each chapter you are provided with a brief outline of practical information, tips, and hints that are intended to supplement your visualization program. When used in conjunction with visualization, it will help you eliminate your negative lifestyle.

These helpful hints for coping with everyday stress come from Dr. Hans Selye. He recommends:

1) *Work off stress:* If you are angry or upset, try to let off steam physically. Garden, play tennis, jog, go for a long walk. This gives you a "flight or fight" outlet for distress.

2) *Talk out worries:* It helps to share worry with someone you trust and respect. Sometimes another person can provide a new perspective which is the very solution you need.

3) *Learn to accept things:* If a problem is beyond control, learn to accept the consequences. Don't waste your time and energy to try and change those things that cannot be changed.

4) *Avoid self-medication:* Certain drugs, particularly alcohol, may seem momentarily to eliminate distress. Avoid them completely. Often they are addicting and usually do nothing to reduce the distress.

5) *Get enough sleep:* Sleep has a way of breaking the concentration-distress cycle.

6) *Balance work and play:* Everyone needs a change of pace. Breaking the customary work-habit cycle with recreation can ease distress.

7) *Do something for others:* Distress causes you to focus on yourself and your problems. Concentration on your problems only causes more distress. Attention directed to others minimizes distress.

8) *Take one thing at a time:* A sure way to be overwhelmed by problems is to try to tackle all of them at one time. By dealing with them one at a time, you have a better chance of solving them.

9) *Give in once in a while:* Admit and recognize when you are wrong and others are right. It is not a crime to be wrong. When you admit it, the distress will fly away.

10) *Make yourself available:* Distress often leads to boredom or a feeling of being left out. Mix with people. Include yourself somewhere.

6. HOW TO EAT, DRINK, AND BE HEALTHY

"You are what you eat."

The majority of people in this country are malnourished. Sound ridiculous or preposterous? It's true. It doesn't matter if you are part of a poverty-income family or an affluent, high-income family—you have equal chances of suffering from malnutrition. This requires a word of explanation because traditionally we have always equated malnutrition with starvation or lack of food. Indeed, this is one of the causes, but in recent years the definition has been expanded. *Malnutrition is the* **lack, imbalance,** *or* **excess** *of one or more of a number of nutrients that are required by the body.* According to today's definition, then, malnourishment is caused by the wrong kinds and quantities of food as well as not enough.

When I am lecturing on wellness, I find most people have some difficulty in grasping the fact that they can have a full stomach three times a day and still be malnourished. The concept of malnutrition as the wrong kind of food has come about because of changes in our eating habits. In years past, the average diet was high in vegetables, fruits, cereals, and breads. For many, meat was a luxury. During the past several generations, we have gotten away from the basics and have developed dietary preferences for meat, eggs, dairy products, and especially "junk foods."

In addition to a shift in taste preference, other factors have been involved in changing dietary patterns. Today over 50 percent of the women work outside the home. The working woman usually does not have the luxury of time to prepare meals. Often, by necessity, it's something from the freezer or a can into the microwave and on the table in thirty minutes. Thirty years ago fast food chain restaurants which deep-fry everything were few. Coin machines filled with salt-covered, high-fat snacks were not on every corner. Because of busy schedules, many view mealtime as a "let's get it over with" exercise instead of the family institution it once was.

These are just a few of the many factors that have been involved in our changing patterns of eating and diet. These changes have been slow in occurring, but they have been cumulative. Let's look at some of the implications of all this.

In the United States, poor diet is one of the most prevalent factors involved in causing premature death. I once saw a poster in a large San Francisco hospital which said that every year tens of thousands of Americans are "eating themselves into an early grave." Are you in this group? Are you placing a limit on your own life-span?

Below are several statements that have been made by the American Heart Association:

> If people curbed their salt intake and didn't smoke, the yearly deaths due to strokes—183,000—would be cut significantly.
>
> If people cut down on the consumption of animal fat, exercised more, and didn't smoke, the annual death rate from heart attacks—638,000—would be considerably decreased.
>
> Improper diet is a prime factor in promoting serious illness and premature deaths. Yearly consumption of sugar in this country is 120 pounds per capita. This carbohydrate intake contributes to obesity and hypoglycemia and increases blood clotting tendencies which can lead to coronary thrombosis.

With this kind of information available, why is dietary malnourishment so rampant in this country? The answer is simple. For most, *dietary habits are established from the satisfaction and pleasure food or drink provides, with little or no consideration for real nutritional value.* Over a period of time, tastes have become accustomed to certain foods and drinks. Unfortunately, in light of information developed during recent years, some of these, when consumed in excess, are harmful.

Why is it that people have such a marked lack of accurate information about proper nutrition? There are a number of reasons. For many, reading and studying about nutrition is not very exciting. Most people can think about a thousand reasons not to take the time and expend the energy to learn about proper nutrition. Second, over the years our tastes have been developed to crave foods which, unknown to us, cause premature death. It is difficult to become motivated, to become knowledgeable about a subject that will require us to give up or reduce consumption of certain foods and drinks to which we have grown pleasantly accustomed. Third, we are surrounded by unbelievably attractive, convincing, and tempting advertising which seduces us to consume food and drink with little or no thought given to the nutritional damage they cause to vital organs and body systems. Such food and drink advertising is designed to start the gastric juices flowing and the appetite to sharpen without reflecting on the fat, cholesterol, sugar, fiber, salt, and preservatives content.

If you are like most, you lack sufficient information about *how* and *why* eating certain foods and drinks destroys body organs and inhibits body systems. Your mind is sending signals to your body saying that any kind or type food you crave is okay. Your desire for food and drink selection is totally uncontrolled. At the present time, your only regulator of control is based upon your personal evaluation: Do I like it? If so, I will eat it (or drink it). If not, I won't. Your consumption of food is based upon the momentary pleasure it gives you without regard to the years it subtracts from your life and the degree to which it destroys high-quality life.

After you have become informed and educated, your mind will send a new set of signals to your body. These new signals will indicate that certain food and drink should be reduced or eliminated from your diet. These foods or drinks will become distasteful and your appetite for them will be lost. When you reach this point, you have achieved one of the most important goals of your life: You have created a mind-body rapport that has your body regulators set to accept only those foods and drinks which are healthful.

Before considering the basic information that you need to start down the road to high-level wellness through proper nutrition, let me emphasize that I am not a nutritional extremist. I am not carried away with organic foods. I do not advocate abstinence from any food or drink. I do not recommend "mega-doses" of dozens of vitamins. I do not condemn or encourage vegetarianism. The reason I do not insist upon extremes in dietary habits is because usually they are impractical, and anything that is impractical is impossible for many. I want to provide you with a nutritional program that can be followed—one that will place you in the top echelon of ideal nutrition.

The program that I will outline for you is based upon moderation. It is a program that will allow you to immediately eliminate or reduce those factors in your diet which are most harmful. From a practical point of view, it is impossible to consume the "ideal" diet. So, let's understand from the beginning that elimination of the unhealthy side of your diet is best, but moderation is better than no change at all.

FATS, PROTEINS, AND CARBOHYDRATES

We are taught early in life that for proper nutrition we must consume a *balanced* diet of fats, proteins, and carbohydrates. There is no question that all three components are necessary for the best possible cellular maintenance, growth, and reproduction. The big question is: What is the ideal balance or ratio?

In the United States, we obtain our calories from the following sources:

fats	42.5 percent
proteins	15.0 percent
carbohydrates	42.5 percent

Since the turn of the century, we have seen an increase in fat consumption and a decrease in carbohydrate intake. This has been caused by eating decreasing amounts of cereals, breads, vegetables, fruits, and more fat-rich meat, eggs, and dairy products.

When considering the different populations of the world, many consume a diet with less than 15 percent fat. The American diet is one of the world's highest in fats. It has required considerable dietary gymnastics on the part of Americans to drive fat consumption up to or above 40 percent of caloric intake. No known food contains 40 percent fat.

Wild animals are made up of a maximum of 10 percent fat. Domesticated animals (cows, pigs, lambs) at most are 15 percent fat. Fruits, vegetables, and grain contain a much smaller percentage of fat. Thus, the average American has, by design, developed a diet that includes concentrated amounts of fat. For many, today's diet emphasizes well-marbled steaks, sausage, bacon, processed foods like hot dogs and cold cuts (which have fat added), butter, cheese, and other dairy products. We have come to love deep-fried foods. Often this can double the fat content.

What is the ideal amount of fat for your diet? While there are many answers to the question, ranging from 10 percent to 30 percent, almost every expert agrees that the current 40-plus percent consumption is too high. Since you will be making a concentrated effort to reduce fat consumption, let's take a more detailed look.

Fats

From a nutritional point of view, fats can be considered saturated or unsaturated. Usually, saturated fats are animal in origin and sold at room temperature (lard, butter). Unsaturated fats are plant in origin and liquid at room temperature (corn oil, peanut oil). Generally, saturated fats are high in cholesterol. Unsaturated fats are lower in cholesterol but may be higher in triglycerides. I find many people are confused about triglycerides and cholesterol. They are not the same, even though elevated levels in the blood of either or both are harmful. Triglycerides are compounds containing three fatty acids. When broken down, the free fatty acids are released into the blood. The amount of triglycerides in the blood can be determined by a laboratory blood test and is an indication of the level of free fatty acids present. Only your physician can order this test. He or she can tell you if your triglyceride level is excessive.

For the sake of simplicity, when we refer to fats we include triglycerides and other fat products. Because of its unique nature, cholesterol will be considered separately.

Numerous studies have shown that ingested fats enter the blood quickly. When individuals drink heavy cream after an overnight fast, the plasma of the blood turns cloudy within a matter of hours. This turbulence of the plasma is due to a buildup of excessive fats. This accumulation of fat in the blood can have a number of harmful effects.

The red cells and platelets (formed elements) in the blood become coated with a thin layer of fat which causes them to become sticky and adhere to each other. This sludging of the formed elements of the blood is illustrated below.

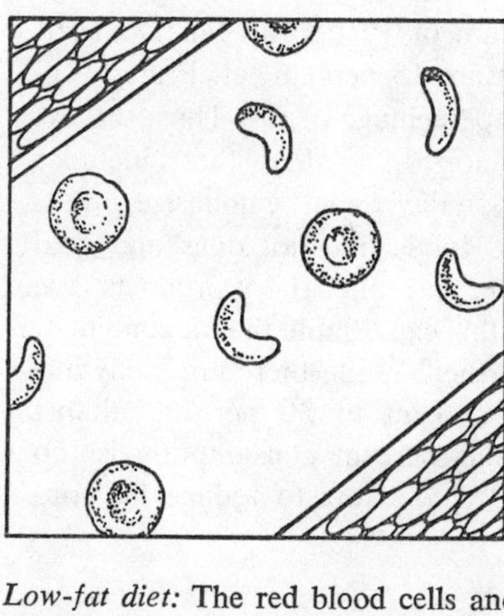

Low-fat diet: The red blood cells and the platelets are clean and free-moving.

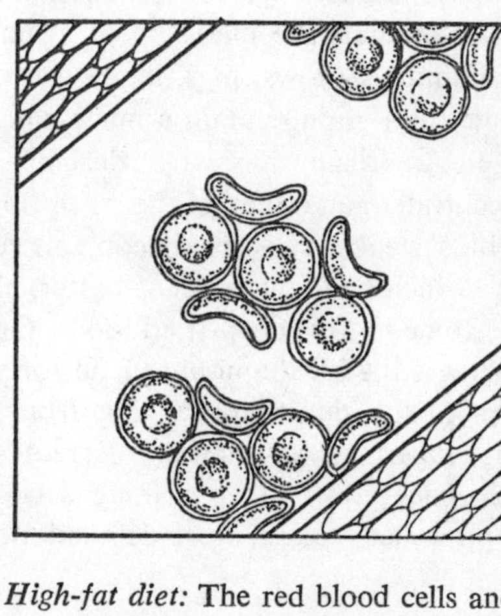

High-fat diet: The red blood cells and the platelets are fat-coated and clumping together.

On the left is a normal distribution of red blood cells and platelets. On the right is what happens after you have eaten a meal that is high in fat content. As these formed elements of the blood clump together, blood flow is reduced. This means that the amount of oxygen available to the brain and cells of the body is diminished following fat intake. Do you doubt it occurs? Think about this. What often happens after a large Thanksgiving Day dinner (usually high in fats)? Have you ever had the urge for a nap on the sofa? If you are like most, the answer is yes. The reason you get sleepy is that your red blood cells and platelets clump together. Because of reduction in blood flow, oxygen to the brain is reduced and the sleepy feeling comes over you. If you further reduce oxygen supply by smoking several cigarettes before and after the meal and have a few Bloody Marys or wine with the meal, the oxygen deficit to the brain is exaggerated. Falling asleep during the first quarter of the football game is inevitable.

Most experts agree that excessive amounts of free fatty acids in the blood (result of elevated triglyceride levels) play a major role in the development of atherosclerosis. Elevated blood cholesterol (discussed later) is also involved. Atherosclerosis is influenced by a number of factors. Heredity seems to be involved. If one or both parents had atherosclerosis, the chance you will develop it is greater than if neither did. Some degree of atherosclerosis can be expected due to the aging process.

If you consume a diet high in fats, you are speeding the onslaught of atherosclerosis. If you restrict fat intake, you are reducing your chance to as near zero as is possible.

Another problem with excessive fats in the diet is that they contain over twice the number of calories per gram as carbohydrates and proteins. Fat contains nine (9) calories per gram as compared with four (4) calories per gram of carbohydrate (including sugar) and protein. Fats usually do not have the "filling" bulk found in carbohydrates and proteins. For this reason, there may be a tendency to want to overconsume foods high in fats. Because of this concentration of calories, there is the inevitable problem of obesity.

Some are of the opinion that elevated levels of fat in the blood can aggravate a preexisting diabetic condition and that latent diabetes can become symptomatic.

So, what is the ideal amount of fat in your daily diet? If you are average, 40 to 45 percent of your calories are from fat. *This must be reduced.* What you must do, starting today, is to become aware of foods and beverages that are high in fats, particularly animal fats. Monitor these foods and beverages carefully. It will be impossible to eliminate them, but you must expend maximum effort to reduce the amount of fat consumed each day. A formula and chart to help you achieve this can be found at the end of this chapter.

Following is a partial list of foods that should be eliminated or restricted because of high-fat content:

avocados
bacon, sausage, ham
gravy mixes and cream sauces
ice cream

beef stew (canned)
butter, margarine, solid shortening
cheese made from whole milk
chicken skin and fat
chips (potato, corn), tortillas
coconut
commercial bread, cornbread, waffles, pancakes, and muffin mixes
corned beef and pastrami
frozen/packages casseroles or dinners
luncheon meat (cold cuts, bologna, salami), hot dogs
mayonnaise
meat high in fat or marbled (beef, lamb, pork)
meat (canned)
milk (whole, chocolate, buttermilk)
nuts (all kinds)
oils (corn, olive, peanut, soybean, cottonseed, safflower)
pastries: cakes, cookies, doughnuts, pies

And above all, avoid any and all deep-fried foods. Remember, fat content of certain foods can double when they are boiled in oil. Now that you have seen the fat "forbidden" list, you are probably wondering what's left. Actually your low-fat diet is very flexible. Following is an abbreviated list of foods that can be eaten while maintaining acceptable fat intake:

bread (dark, whole grain)
cereals and grains
chicken and turkey (skin removed)
fish
fruits
fruit juices
skim milk
vegetables

At the end of this chapter there is an expanded list of foods and beverages that you should eat and the reasons why.

The main point about fat consumption is to monitor and eliminate or restrict those foods known to be high in fat content. If this is done you will probably cut your fat intake by 50 percent. You will find you can quickly readjust your eating habits and kick the high-fat habit with a minimum of difficulty.

Cholesterol

Much controversy and, indeed, mysticism surrounds the subject of cholesterol. Recent studies have suggested that cholesterol covers the gamut—all the way from being good for you to being the prime cause of cardiovascular diseases. I would like to approach this seemingly confusing subject from the standpoint of what we know for sure about cholesterol.

Many are under the impression that cholesterol is a fat. This is easy to understand since it is almost always discussed along with fats. Actually, cholesterol is a waxy, insoluble material which is a sterol—a steroid-like compound.

Cholesterol itself is not harmful. In fact, cholesterol is a naturally occurring substance found in virtually every cell of the body and produced primarily by the liver. It is a necessity for certain body functions. Cholesterol is responsible for the production of certain enzymes that are required for proper digestion. In the female, cholesterol is the forerunner of certain hormones, particularly progesterone-like hormones. From this it can be seen that the blanket charge that "cholesterol is harmful" is not true. A certain level of cholesterol in the body is not only normal but necessary.

What is harmful is when the amount of cholesterol in the blood rises above certain levels. There is no controversy that an elevated level of cholesterol in the blood is harmful and is a major factor in causing atherosclerosis. This is the buildup of foreign materials on the inner walls of the arteries. In addition to cholesterol, triglycerides, plaque, and cellular debris are involved.

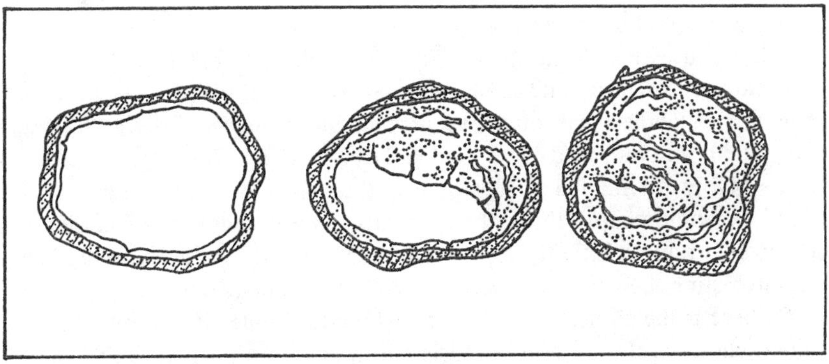

Atherosclerosis

Pictured above is a cross section of three arteries. On the left is a healthy artery, which is free of atherosclerosis. It can be seen that the internal diameter is large, allowing the maximum amount of blood to pass through. In the middle is a mild case of atherosclerosis. The buildup of cholesterol and other materials is beginning. Blood flow is starting to be reduced. On the right is advanced atherosclerosis with the blood flow drastically curtailed. The internal diameter of the artery is only a fraction of what it should be. Blood flow is down to a trickle. In this situation, it is easy for a blood clot to form. If this occurs in a coronary artery, the result is a heart attack.

What is a normal level of cholesterol in the blood? Even here there is no agreement. Depending upon the reference, below are listed upper limits of normal:

300 mg. per 100 milliliters
225 mg. per 100 milliliters
100 plus your age mg. per 100 milliliters

The only person who can tell what your blood cholesterol should be and if it is above normal is your physician. Ask your physician for the information. If you are interested in high-level nutritional wellness, you must know if your blood cholesterol is above normal. If it is, you may be consciously and knowingly contributing to your own atherosclerosis.

From a practical point of view, what does elevated blood cholesterol really mean? The American Heart Association has stated that a person (man) with a blood cholesterol of 250 mg. or more has a *three*-times greater risk of having a heart attack than a person with a blood cholesterol of 194 mg. or less. Nothing else really needs to be said. Elevated blood cholesterol causes the arteries to age prematurely. This speeded-up aging is called atherosclerosis.

What causes an elevation in your blood cholesterol? Is it based upon the cholesterol you eat? Not necessarily. Some people can eat huge amounts of cholesterol and have normal blood levels. Others can ingest only small amounts and have extremely high levels. Why is this? It seems to be involved with the liver, which is the prime site for cholesterol production. Some people think that if you eat large amounts of cholesterol, the liver produces little. If you eat little or none, it produces more. This is an interesting theory and is, perhaps, valid for some people.

So here is the cholesterol controversy made simple. If you monitor your blood cholesterol on a regular basis and it is within normal limits, there is no need to restrict cholesterol intake. If it's high, then intake must be limited. This is the scientific approach. The only problem is that most people do not and will not monitor blood cholesterol. This, then, leads to the practical approach to the gigantic problem of cholesterol and atherosclerosis. *If you are not sure of blood cholesterol levels, be on the safe side and restrict cholesterol intake!* Remember the old saying, "Better safe than sorry."

How do you go about restricting cholesterol intake? It's not as complicated as it may seem because there are only a few food groups that are excessively high in cholesterol content. They are organ meat, red meat, shellfish, cheese, eggs, and butter. Below is listed the approximate cholesterol content for these foods based upon a four-ounce portion:

CHOLESTEROL CONTENT OF VARIOUS FOODS
(4-ounce portion)

Organ meats		*Meat*	
Kidney	375 mg.	Veal	90 mg.
Brains	2,000 mg.	Pork	70 mg.
Heart	150 mg.	Beef	70 mg.
Liver	300 mg.	Lamb	70 mg.
Sweetbreads	250 mg.	*Cheese*	
Shellfish		Cheddar	100 mg.
Crab	125 mg.	Cream	120 mg.
Shrimp	125 mg.	*Butter*	250 mg.
Oysters	200 mg.		
Lobster	200 mg.	*Eggs*	
		(2 eggs, yolk & white)	500 mg.

At the present time, it is estimated that the average intake of cholesterol is slightly over 1,000 milligrams daily. This level of intake is, in part, responsible for the fact that the majority of deaths in the United States are caused by cardiovascular diseases. Some authorities are now recommending that cholesterol consumption be reduced to around 300 mg. per day.

So if, in the achievement of your own self-responsibility for high-level wellness, you determine to limit your intake of cholesterol, what should you do? Limit the number of eggs you eat. One egg yoke contains 250 milligrams of cholesterol. Be aware of all the foods containing invisible eggs (egg noodles, bakery products, puddings, mayonnaise, etc.). You should limit the amount of organ meats. Shellfish are high in cholesterol. All red meat must be curtailed, along with cheeses, and butter.

LIPOPROTEINS

As indicated, cholesterol is a water-insoluble waxy substance. Since it is not dissolved in the blood, it must have a special method of transport through the body. This is accomplished by the lipoproteins. There are several lipoproteins, but two have received a tremendous amount of publicity lately. They are high-density lipoprotein (HDL) and low-density lipoprotein (LDL). Some feel that HDL and LDL are more important than cholesterol itself in causing or preventing atherosclerosis.

HDL and LDL attach to the cholesterol and act like a trailer truck. They move cholesterol through the body. There is one major difference between HDL and LDL; namely, they always move in opposite directions. The LDL is the transportation system that picks up fresh cholesterol at the point of manufacture (liver) and distributes it throughout the circulatory system. As the LDL-cholesterol circulates around the arteries, certain amounts are deposited on the inner walls. This can produce atherosclerosis. Needless to say, this spread of cholesterol by LDL is not good.

On the other hand, HDL does just the opposite. It travels through the circulatory system collecting cholesterol and always moves toward the liver. Since the liver is the organ of metabolism, this is where the cholesterol is destroyed and prepared for excretion. Some have referred to HDL as the "cholesterol scavenger." In this melodrama of the lipoproteins, LDL is the bad guy wearing the black hat, while HDL is the hero on the white horse.

Below is an illustration depicting the role of LDL and HDL in the pickup and delivery of cholesterol through the circulatory system.

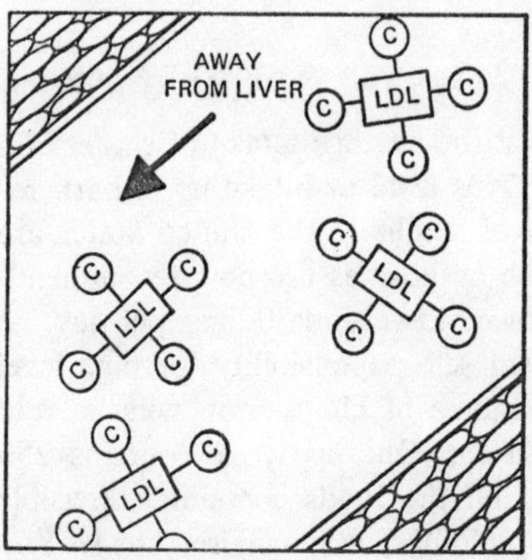

LDL: Picking up cholesterol from the liver and distributing it throughout the body.

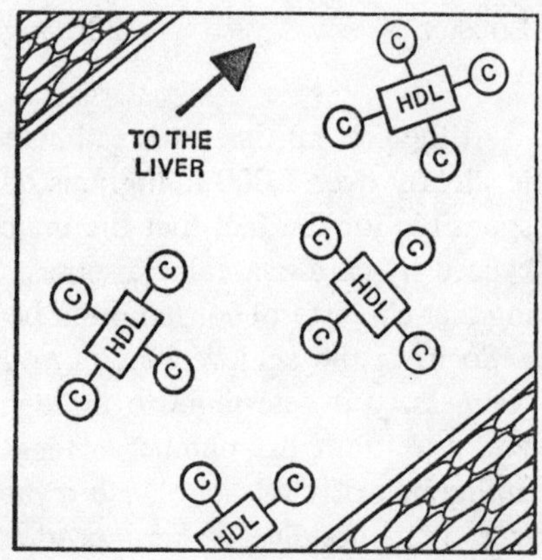

HDL: The cholesterol scavenger gathering cholesterol and carrying it to the liver for metabolism and excretion.

On the left is the LDL-cholesterol complex moving away from the liver. On the right, it can be seen that the HDL-cholesterol always moves in the opposite direction.

From this, it appears that what you are looking for in order to achieve high-level nutritional wellness is a high level of HDL. Right? Not necessarily so. I am told that one of the "in" things now is to be able to intelligently discuss your HDL level, but I caution you that this, in itself, is not the whole story. What you should be interested in is the *ratio* between your LDL and HDL. To have a very high level of HDL along with a high level of LDL accomplishes little. The goal is for you to be able to develop a program that will increase your HDL and decrease your LDL.

The determination of your LDL and HDL levels can be accomplished only by your physician with a laboratory blood test. The test usually is expensive, beyond what some can or will pay, so let's look at the LDL-HDL story from the standpoint of what has been learned from study groups.

A newborn baby has a one-to-one ratio of LDL and HDL. For the majority of people, by the time they become adults, the ratio is 4–6 to one. Four to six times more LDL than HDL! What causes this change? Some studies have suggested that the causes are smoking, obesity, and the sedentary life.

When people stop smoking, lose weight, and become involved in a regular exercise program, HDL usually goes up and LDL goes down. As a group, marathon runners usually have the highest HDL ratios. Heredity is also involved. When families have been studied which enjoy extremely long life-spans, the results have been uniform: high HDL and low LDL.

In summary, you may want to have your physician determine your LDL-HDL levels. That's fine. If it's impossible or impractical, you can probably be successful in changing your 4–6 to one ratio by becoming involved in a program of regular, sustained exercise and by eliminating the two negative lifestyles—if you have them—smoking and obesity. The end result can reduce the possibility of atherosclerosis and the chance of stroke and heart attack.

Proteins

Proteins are made up of building units called amino acids. Amino acids are required by people of all ages to replace tissues that are constantly being broken down. There are twenty-two amino acids, of which nine are called essential. The essential amino acids are those that cannot be manufactured by the body and must come from the diet.

Proteins are important to the diet because of the following roles they have in good nutrition:

Maintenance and growth

Chief solid matter of muscle, organs, and endocrine glands; matrix of bone, teeth, skin, nails, hair, blood cells, and serum. First need for amino acids is to supply the materials for the building and continuous replacement of these tissues and fluids throughout life.

Regulation of body process

Body proteins have highly specialized functions in the regulation of body processes. For example, hemoglobin, the oxygen-carrying component of the red blood cells, is a protein. The body's defense mechanism, the antibodies, are protein in nature. Many enzymes are protein. Numerous hormones such as insulin, epinephrine, and thyroid hormone are protein-like.

Energy

Body proteins can be used for energy. However, this is not desirable. Energy needs should come from carbohydrates. In the absence of adequate amounts of carbohydrates, proteins are used to supply energy. These protein supplies may come from the diet or body storage. In either case, it is not desirable because adequate protein may not be available for synthesis and to regulate body processes.

In the United States, approximately 15 percent of total calories come from protein. According to most authorities, this is the ideal amount that is adequate for the continuous synthesis of new protein tissue throughout the body.

Much has been said and written about high-protein/no-carbohydrate diets. The theory behind all of them is to eliminate or nearly eliminate carbohydrates from the diet. Carbohydrates are the body's first choice for energy production. If carbohydrates are not present, the body turns on its own protein and fat for energy. The protein in muscles (including heart muscle), glands, and components of the blood are broken down and converted to energy. Obviously this is not a healthy situation. The idea behind the liquid-protein/no-carbohydrate or animal-protein/no-carbohydrate diets is to eat or drink enough protein to satisfy the body's need for energy. This is called by some a "protein sparing" effect.

Following are two illustrations that point out why carbohydrate conversion to energy is preferred to protein conversion to energy.

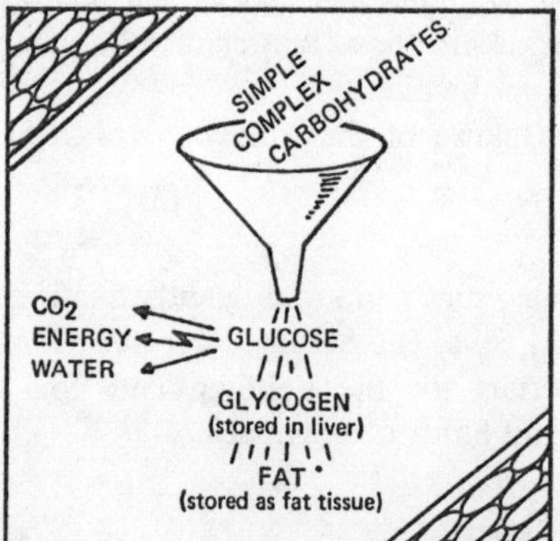

Energy from carbohydrates: The reaction is clean, with no toxic by-products.

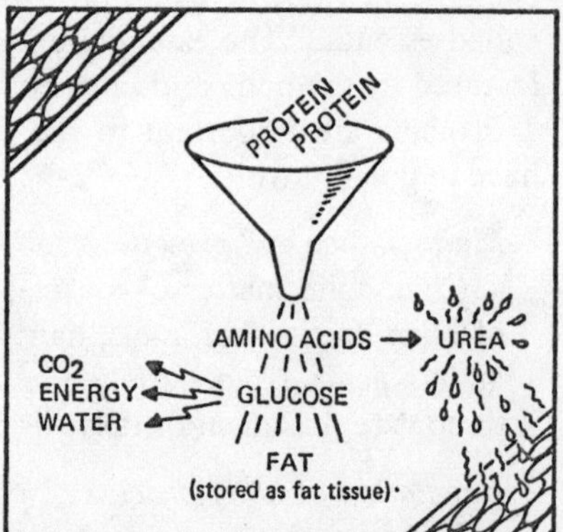

Energy from protein: Conversion requires an extra step and produces urea, which is toxic.

On the left is carbohydrate conversion. This is the cleanest and most efficient. Simple and complex carbohydrates are metabolized to glucose, which results in energy, carbon dioxide, and water. When adequate energy is available, the excess glucose is stored in the form of glycogen and fat. On the right where ingested protein is being broken down, you can see the big difference between how carbohydrates and protein yield energy. When protein is used, an extra step is required. The protein must be converted to amino acids of which about half are turned into glucose and half into fatty acids. This breakdown of amino acids results in a buildup of urea which is toxic and must be neutralized. This is accomplished by attracting water to it. This causes excessive body water loss and explains why when you go on a high-protein/no-carbohydrate diet, large amounts of "weight" are lost very quickly. Actually it is only water loss, which is gained back when the diet returns to normal. This clearly illustrates why carbohydrates should be the prime source of energy.

Proteins are found in a variety of foods. For the sake of simplicity these can be broken down into three groups, those which are high, medium, and low in protein content.

HIGH	MEDIUM	LOW
dry milk	legumes	fruits
meat	flour	vegetables
fish	cereals	
poultry	liquid milk	
cheese		
nuts		
eggs		

This chart has nothing to do with suggesting which protein food source is preferred. It concerns only concentration.

There have been definite shifts in the source of dietary protein since the first of the century. Sixty years ago, we obtained 38 percent of our protein from flour and cereal products. Today it is 18 percent. During the same period, red meat as a source of protein has gone from 25 percent to 32 percent. Today we obtain 70 percent of our total protein from nonplant sources (meat, poultry, fish, dairy products, and eggs).

The basic problem, which is beginning to be recognized, is that many of the sources of animal protein are also the highest in fats and cholesterol. This is causing a serious examination and re-evaluation of the non-animal sources of protein.

The question that comes up often when considering non-animal protein is: Is it safe and adequate for proper nutrition? It must be realized that the majority of the world's population live on diets in which protein is derived solely from plants and are very healthy. Animal sources of protein are either not available or too expensive. Usually, the plants used to supply protein are legumes, whole grains, nuts, and vegetables. Some of the food usually used in these low-meat societies are corn, beans, peas, rice, bread, and grain cereals. Numerous studies have pointed out that this diet provides more than adequate amounts of amino acids.

Approximately 15 percent of your calories should come from protein. The average American is consuming about the right amount of protein; the problem is in the source of protein. We need to *shift the emphasis away from animal protein, which is high in fat and cholesterol, and increase non-animal protein.* This will accomplish the following:

- Maintain protein at the present level.
- Reduce the amounts of animal fat and cholesterol.
- Increase the amount of fiber in the diet.
- Provide greater food bulk with no increase in calories (perhaps a reduction).

In summary, when you consider protein, you must get away from the traditional thinking that the only source of protein is eggs, red meat, milk, and cheese. You can get abundant protein in fish, chicken, turkey, fruits, vegetables, bread, and grain cereals. A part of becoming informed and on your way to high-level nutritional wellness is to realize that plant proteins do exist and can provide a good portion of your protein requirements.

Carbohydrates

Throughout the generations, carbohydrates have been praised and condemned. Based upon whatever the current fad, we have been told that we should be on a high-carbohydrate diet or a low-carbohydrate diet. Where should carbohydrates fit in the nutritional puzzle of high-level wellness?

Let's consider a few facts. First, we need carbohydrates. All forms of carbohydrates are ultimately converted to glucose. Glucose is utilized by the cells of the body for energy. It is the only food for the brain. Twenty-five percent of total body glucose is consumed by the brain.

When considering the different forms of carbohydrates, they can be divided into two basic groups, the *simple* and the *complex.* Simple carbohydrates are the monosaccharides and disaccharides, and they are represented by table sugar, brown sugar, syrups, and honey. Complex carbohydrates are the polysaccharides, which are referred to as starches. Fruits, vegetables, and grains are high in complex carbohydrates.

One of the basic differences between simple and complex carbohydrates is in regard to their digestion and absorption. The simple carbohydrates require little or no digestion and deliver to the blood rapid and erratic amounts of glucose. On the other hand, the complex carbohydrates are broken down more slowly and the end product—glucose—is passed into the blood in a slow, smooth, and constant way.

Following are illustrations of the differences between simple and complex carbohydrates in regard to delivery of glucose to the blood.

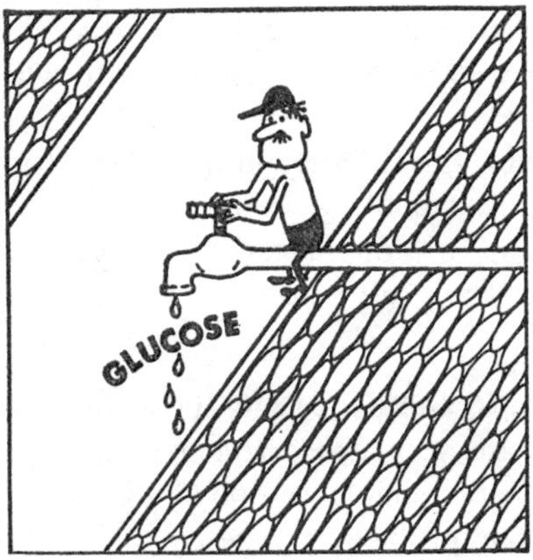

Complex carbohydrates: Glucose is delivered to the blood in a smooth and continuous way.

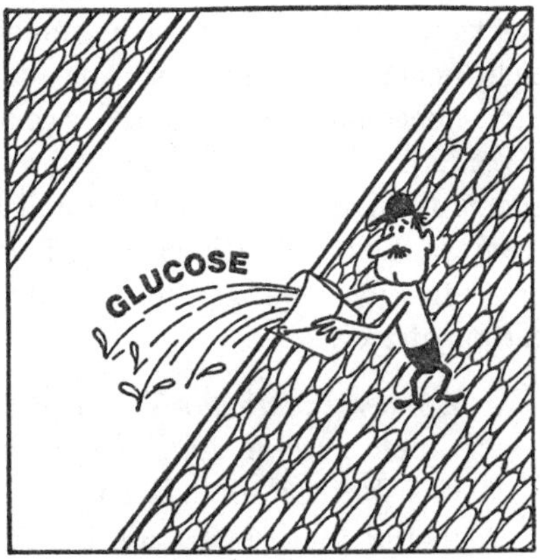

Simple carbohydrates: Large amounts of glucose are dumped into the blood in erratic loads.

On the left is Mr. Complex Carbohydrate delivering a slow, continuous supply of glucose. On the right is Mr. Simple Carbohydrate dumping large amounts of glucose periodically as the bucket becomes full.

Because of the rapid digestion and absorption of the simple carbohydrates, blood sugar patterns can fluctuate. Since simple carbohydrates are digested and absorbed faster, the feeling of hunger occurs sooner and more frequently. Lastly, simple carbohydrates have no nutritional value and provide no fiber.

The complex carbohydrates are just the opposite. Because of slower digestion and absorption, they result in a more constant flow of glucose into the blood, which is more ideal for brain and cellular consumption. Blood sugar alterations are less likely to occur. Since complex carbohydrates (starches) are found in vegetables, fruits, and grains, vitamins, minerals, and fiber are provided for the body. Because of the slower release of glucose, complex carbohydrates may postpone hunger for longer periods of time. This explains why raw vegetables, fresh fruit, or a slice of plain dark bread make excellent snack items.

From this you can see that for high-level nutritional wellness, simple carbohydrates should be minimized and complex carbohydrates emphasized.

Back at the turn of the century, our average carbohydrate intake was about 30 percent simple carbohydrates and 70 percent complex. By 1975 we were consuming about 55 percent of our carbohydrates as simple sugars and 45 percent as complex starches. One of the reasons for this shift is that we have gotten away from fruits, vegetables, and grains and moved to a diet high in meats. Another factor is our dependency on items like soft drinks. About 23 percent of all the sugar we consume is in soft drinks. In 1960 our average annual consumption of soft drinks was 192 eight-ounce units per person per year. By 1974 this had increased to 430 eight-ounce units per person per year.

As indicated, simple carbohydrates enter immediately into the blood in erratic fashion. This rapid rise and fall in available glucose can cause the many problems associated with fluctuation in blood sugar (hypoglycemia and hyperglycemia). Other potential problems are associated with simple carbohydrates.

- *Concentrated calories* Sugar, syrups, and honey are 100 percent simple carbohydrate and as such are very *concentrated* in calories. Because of this concentration, the simple carbohydrates are one of the prime reasons behind our problem of obesity. Simple carbohydrates are often called "empty calories" because they have no nutritional value—no vitamins, minerals, or fiber.
- *Dental cavities* All carbohydrates are harmful to the teeth because they provide a favorable environment for the rapid growth of bacteria. Simple carbohydrates (sticky candy and other sweets) are most harmful because of the concentrated amount of sugar they place on the surface of the teeth.
- *Blood fats* All carbohydrates will cause an elevation in blood fats, but it is more evident when simple carbohydrates are eaten. Studies have shown that when people switch from a complex to a simple carbohydrate diet, blood fats go up significantly.
- *Gastrointestinal irritation* Simple carbohydrates can cause irritation of the inner lining of the gastrointestinal tract. This can lead to distension, flatulence, and diarrhea.

In the past, many people have thought of carbohydrates as that part of the diet to be avoided because they cause weight gain.

If you have this attitude, it must change. Recognize carbohydrates for what they are—a real Dr. Jekyll and Mr. Hyde, the schizophrenic of the nutritional world. Recognize and become informed about the two different kinds. You must *recognize* simple carbohydrates as harmful and that they are to be eliminated from the diet. Complex carbohydrates are beneficial and to be increased.

What you must do is try to eliminate sugar, syrups, and honey.

Remember, 75 percent of the simple carbohydrates we consume are "invisible," that is, they are not coming from the sugar bowl and the syrup pitcher. Be aware of the 75 percent used in cooking and food preparation. I know that total elimination of these products is impossible, but an attempt at elimination will result in maximum reduction.

Since carbohydrates are required for energy, you will offset the reduction in simple carbohydrates with a definite increase in complex carbohydrates. Foods high in complex carbohydrates are:

- *All vegetables* Particularly good for you are rice, potatoes, peas, beans, corn, green and yellow vegetables.
- *Fruits* The best are those with edible skins, such as apples, pears, plums, etc.
- *Bread* Eat dark bread made with unrefined or whole-grain flour.
- *Pasta* In addition to the regular, try whole-wheat (avoid high egg content).

Does it sound strange that someone recommends that you *eat* potatoes, bread, and pasta? We have always been educated that they were at the top of the forbidden list. They were "too fattening." Let's look at a few facts. A medium-sized baked potato contains about the same number of calories as the "nonfattening" apple. It's what we do to the potato that can make it high-calorie. When you cut the potato and subject it to five minutes in boiling fat, the caloric content *doubles.* When you take the low-calorie baked potato and heap on butter, cheese, and sour cream, you double or triple the calories. Learn to eat your potatoes baked and plain—they're delicious. If you feel you must have a topping, try low-fat yogurt. You will have difficulty telling it from sour cream. A similar situation exists with bread. A slice of bread contains about 70 calories. Provided that it is not white bread, there is no other way you can get the nutritional value, fiber, and full feeling from just 70 calories.

So, in summary, you should increase your overall consumption of carbohydrates with a decrease in the simple and a sharp increase in the complex carbohydrates. This recommendation will provide a diet closer to those of a number of cultures in the world where cardiovascular and metabolic diseases are low. It puts us closer to the diet we ate around the turn of the century, when the consumption of vegetables, fruits, and grain foods was high and the consumption of meat, eggs, and dairy products was low. The readjustment of your carbohydrate intake is an important part of achieving high-level nutritional wellness.

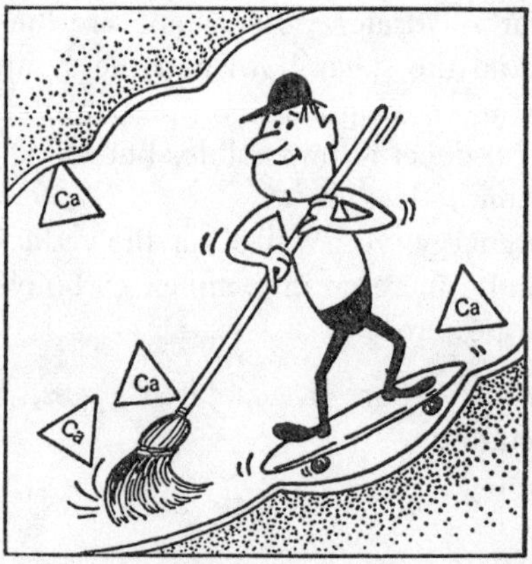

High-fiber diet: Waste material moves through the bowel faster, carrying cancer toxins out of the body.

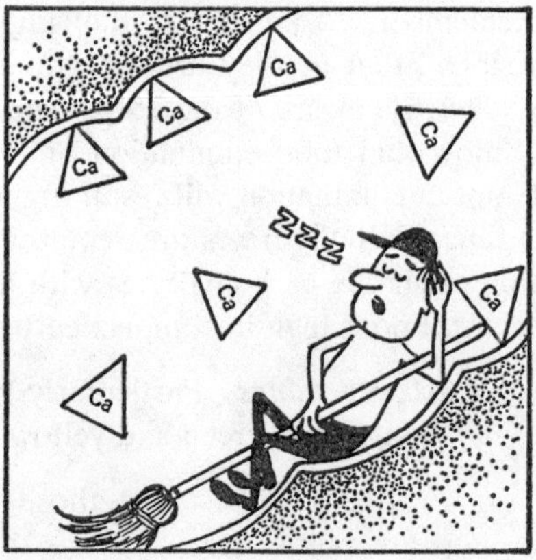

Low-fiber diet: There is little or no bulk to waste material. It moves through the bowel slowly, leaving cancer toxins in the body.

FIBER

I read an article a short while ago which stated, "It used to be 'carbohydrate.' Then it was 'cholesterol' and 'saturated fats.' The food-word for the 1980s is 'fiber.'" It is not true that interest in carbohydrates, cholesterol, and saturated fats is low, but I do agree that increasing attention should be given to the role of fiber in our diet.

Where has fiber been all these years? It's been with us, but not in the limelight. We have always heard about "roughage" or "bulk" foods that were good (according to the cereal advertisements) to prevent "irregularity." That is, in fact, one of the actions of fiber. Certain foods such as fruits, vegetables, whole grains, bran cereals, nuts, and seeds are not completely digested. This undigested portion increases the bulk of waste material and results in regular, productive, distress-free trips to the bathroom.

On the other hand, if the diet is high in foods that are fiber-free (steaks, chops, cakes, cheese, ice cream, etc.), they are almost totally digested and absorbed. This results in low bulk and slow elimination. The results can be constipation and all its problems.

This "increasing the bulk" characteristic of high-fiber foods has been talked about and understood for a number of years, but recently, more exciting advantages of a high-fiber diet have been described. In countries or cultures where the diet is basically high-fiber, it has been noted that cancer of the large bowel is almost nonexistent. This is attributed to the high-fiber diet. Since the high-fiber diet causes waste material to move

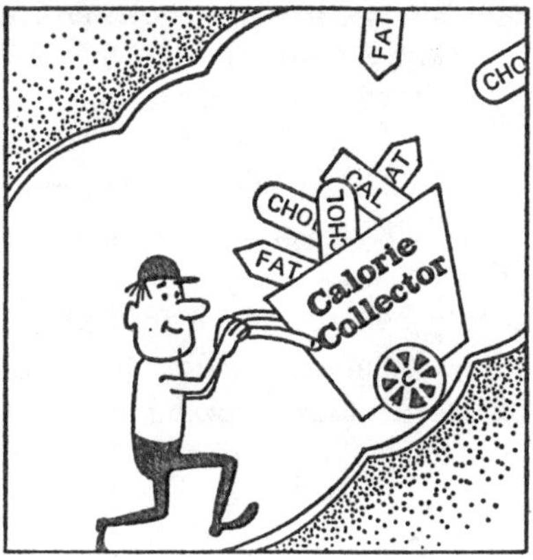

High-fiber diet: Prevents the total absorption of calories, fat, and cholesterol.

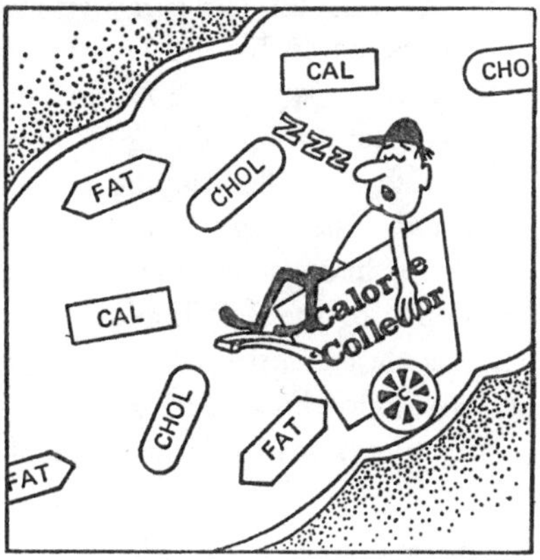

Low-fiber diet: Calories, fat, and cholesterol are completely absorbed.

through faster, the toxins or agents that can cause cancer are eliminated quicker.

On page 112 are two illustrations depicting the difference in high- and low-fiber diets and the role high fiber plays in bowel cancer.

On the left is an illustration representing a high-fiber diet. Waste material is moving through the bowel faster, collecting cancer-causing toxins and carrying them out of the body. On the right is a low-fiber diet illustration. It shows slow movement through the bowel, leaving the cancer toxins undisturbed.

In large population groups that eat a high-fiber diet, cardiovascular diseases—strokes and heart attacks—are very low. The reason for this is that high-fiber foods are almost uniformly low in fats and cholesterol. In addition, it has been suggested that if high-fiber foods are consumed along with high-fat and cholesterol foods, the fiber may prevent the absorption of a portion of the fat and cholesterol.

The high-fiber diet is an absolute "must" for the person who is trying to lose weight. There are a number of reasons for this. First, high-fiber foods are usually lower-calorie than low-fiber foods. Second, the high-fiber diet does have more bulk and is, therefore, more filling. This accomplishes two things: hunger pangs will disappear faster and they will stay away longer. Because of the bulk, there is a tendency to eat slower and have the meal or food last longer. Third, research shows that volunteers on a high-fiber diet excrete more calories as waste than when consuming the same number of calories in low-fiber foods.

Above are illustrations which portray the role of a high-fiber diet in preventing absorption of a portion of calories, fat, and cholesterol. The illustration on the left is a high-fiber diet. Calories, fat, and cholesterol are being collected by the high-fiber and quickly eliminated from the body. On the right is a low-fiber diet moving slowly with all of the calories, fat, and cholesterol remaining for absorption.

A high-fiber diet may be beneficial for the diabetic or diabetes-prone individual. One study has pointed out that diabetics who went on a high-fiber diet had a reduction in insulin requirements.

Stones in the gall bladder are commonly believed to be formed from excess cholesterol in the bile. Studies suggest that adding fiber to the diet reduces bile cholesterol. A University of Bristol study recorded an 80 percent reduction in bile cholesterol when patients were put on a high-fiber diet.

A number of bowel problems may be prevented or minimized by high-fiber. Some of these are diverticulitis and appendicitis.

Since the high-fiber diet has long been neglected and is obviously beneficial for a program of nutritional excellence, what are the best high-fiber foods?

Cereals: cereals marked as being all-bran or high in bran, oatmeal (not instant), shredded wheat

Breads: bread, cakes, muffins, and pastries made with whole-grain flour (whole wheat or whole rye)

Seeds: whole sesame seeds, sunflower seeds, and seed-filled berries such as raspberries and blackberries

Vegetables and Fruits: mangoes, apples, Brussels sprouts, eggplant, cabbage, corn, oranges, peas, green beans, lettuce, pears, onions, celery, cucumbers, tomatoes, cauliflower, bananas, rhubarb, old and new potatoes, turnips

How much fiber do you need? One serving of a bran-containing cereal in the morning is a good way to start. Add a few servings of other high-fiber items from the above list each day and your requirements for fiber will be taken care of.

SALT

A certain amount of salt is required for normal body function. It regulates the passage of water into and out of the cells of the body. It is also involved in the metabolism of carbohydrates and proteins.

The main problem in this country is that we have developed a pro-salt taste which results in the consumption of amounts far greater than

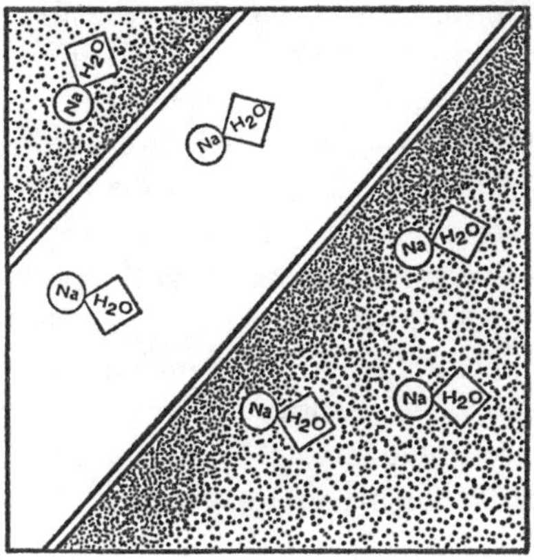

Low-salt diet: The proper amount of sodium for normal body function. No excessive retention of water.

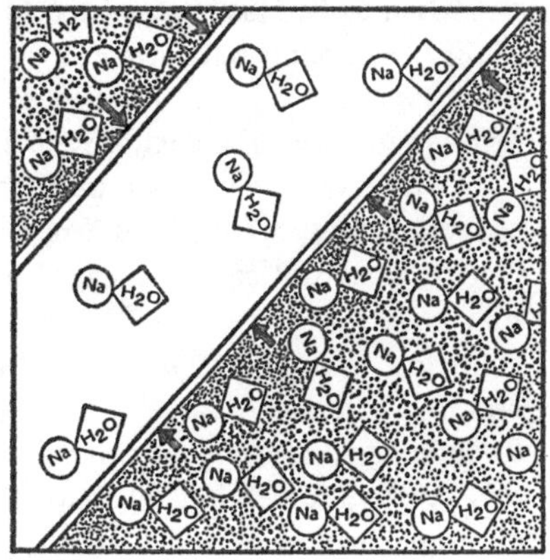

High-salt diet: Excessive sodium in extracellular spaces and in the blood, causing an increase in blood pressure and edema.

needed. Salt is sodium chloride, of which 40 percent is sodium. The commonly accepted minimum daily requirement for sodium is 400 milligrams per day. You get this amount of sodium in 2 ounces of cured ham, 4 ounces of salted peanuts, 4 ounces of brick cheese, or 6 green olives. It is estimated that the average intake of salt in the United States is about 10 grams (4,000 mg. of sodium) daily. *Based on averages, we consume ten times more sodium than is required for normal body function.*

Hypertension

The main problem associated with excessive consumption of salt is hypertension (high blood pressure). It is estimated that 20 percent of the adult population has hypertension. Fifty percent of those with hypertension don't know they have the disease. This is because there are usually no symptoms associated with the problem. Hypertension has been called the "silent killer" because of this unique ability to do tremendous damage to the body without warning signals.

What is hypertension? It is a condition in which the blood is moving through the circulatory system under excessive pressure. It's as if you hooked a garden hose up to a powerful fire truck pumper. You are supposed to use a four-inch hose instead of a half-inch one. When the pump goes into action, it is only a period of time until the garden hose ruptures. The same thing can happen inside the body.

What causes the blood pressure to go up? The arteries and veins are supposed to be elastic and expand with each contraction of the heart. This ability to expand outward keeps the blood pressure constant and normal. Factors such as stress, diet, lack of exercise, worry, and aging cause the arteries to lose this elasticity. When this occurs, blood pressure goes up. Atherosclerosis, which is a narrowing of the inner diameter of the arteries, reduces the space for blood flow and increases blood pressure.

Why does salt cause or aggravate high blood pressure? It is the sodium that causes the problem. When salt is eaten, the sodium (Na) splits off from the chloride (Cl). The sodium quickly finds its way into the blood and then into the extracellular spaces. Elevated levels of sodium in the extracellular spaces are unnatural and are not tolerated by the body. For this reason, something must neutralize the high level of sodium. This is accomplished by water (H_2O). The sodium, like a magnet, attracts the water. The more sodium in the extracellular space, the greater the amount of water attracted. This sodium-water complex expands the volume of the extracellular spaces and places pressure on the arteries.

Pictured on page 115 is a normal amount of sodium in the extracellular space. It is buffered with water, but because the amount of sodium is not high, increased blood pressure is no problem. On the right are excessive amounts of sodium in the extracellular spaces. The sodium has attracted large amounts of water. The extra amount of captive water places pressure on the arteries. In addition, extra sodium in the blood may increase blood volume; thus, the blood pressure increases. The increase in water retention in the extracellular spaces is also responsible for body-wide edema or "bloating."

You may be wondering why hypertension is such a problem. After all, it usually has no symptoms. Hypertension is one of the primary causes of strokes and heart attacks. A stroke can be caused by a clot lodging in an artery and preventing blood flow. It can also be the result of hypertension blowing a hole in an artery. In either case, the end result is lack of blood flow to some part of the body. If it happens to be in the area of the brain, paralysis or death may result. If in the lungs, pulmonary function can be diminished or lost. If it occurs in the heart, a heart attack occurs. In addition, hypertension can lead to congestive heart failure and kidney failure. Many experts consider hypertension the most serious of the cardiovascular risk factors. It is a disease that can lead to catastrophic illness or death.

Nearly everyone is familiar with how you determine blood pressure. A machine is available which measures the pressure of the blood against an artery in the upper arm as the heart contracts and relaxes. These numbers are referred to as the systolic (upper) and diastolic (lower). Much has been written lately about which is more important. Both are important! Normal blood pressure will vary with age. The following are generally accepted normals for men and women.

NORMAL BLOOD PRESSURE

AGE	MEN	WOMEN
6–8 years	100/60	100/60
20–25 years	122/76	116/72
30–35 years	127/80	124/78
40–45 years	132/82	129/80
50–55 years	137/84	134/83
70 and over	146/81	159/85

Individual situations and surroundings can cause your blood pressure to fluctuate.

Hypertension is, perhaps, one of the most prominent influences in causing premature death. The American Heart Association has stated that a person (man) with a systolic pressure over 150 has more than *twice* the risk of a heart attack and nearly *four* times the risk of stroke as has a person (man) with a systolic pressure of 120 or less. I hope you will stop and reflect on this fact. Elevated blood pressure can increase your chance for a stroke *four* times and double the chance for heart attack. Accept the self-responsibility for monitoring your blood pressure. It could mean the difference between life and death.

A part of high-level wellness is for you to assume the responsibility of knowing and monitoring your blood pressure on a regular basis. Regular means taking your blood pressure at least once a month or more often. This is easy to do. You can purchase a good blood pressure machine for a nominal cost. Most fire stations which have paramedics will be pleased to check your blood pressure. There are increasing numbers of machines in shopping centers which will check your blood pressure. (Be sure they are in proper working order.) The purpose of the constant vigil is so that you can be aware of any changes or shifts. If you notice your blood pressure is increasing, immediately go see your physician. He or she will know what to do in order to have your blood pressure back to normal in a short period of time.

One important word of advice. If your physician places you on a low-salt diet for hypertension, do your best to follow the instructions. If you are placed on medication, it is imperative you take it exactly as prescribed. Recent studies have pointed out that individuals who take medication on a regular basis, and those who become informed about how and why hypertension is harmful, decrease the chance of stroke or heart attack. I stress this point because, for many, it is difficult to take medication on a regular basis when there are no symptoms. Don't fall into this trap. Staying on your diet and taking your medication can add years to your life.

One way you can prevent or postpone the occurrence of hypertension is to limit your intake of salt. You might wonder how we can be so sure there is a relationship between salt intake and hypertension. Many studies have been done to prove the point. Below is an example of this work:

NATIONALITY	AVERAGE SALT INTAKE (GRAMS/DAY)	INCIDENCE OF HYPERTENSION
Eskimos	less than 5	less than 10% of population
Americans	10	20% of population
Japanese (northern Japan)	40	45% of population

One of the major problems we have is the "invisible" salt we are subjected to. We consume about 25 percent of our salt from the salt shaker. The rest is in the foods and beverages we eat and drink. You must become familiar with the foods and beverages that are high in salt. The following abbreviated list will help you:

all salted snacks—nuts, chips, pretzels
bacon
baking powder
biscuits—canned
bouillon
brine packed foods—olives, pickles, sauerkraut
butter
cakes
catsup
cereals—most, except bran and wheat
cheese—all kinds
doughnuts
flour—self-rising
frozen dinners and casseroles
margarine
meat—canned
meat, processed—luncheon meat, hot dogs, salami
milk—dry
mustard
peanut butter
salad dressing
sausage
soup and stew—canned or mix
soy sauce
vegetables—canned

All of these foods should be eliminated from your diet. If you find this impossible, reduce consumption as much as possible.

Do you ever salt your food before you taste it? Do you pour salt on out of habit? Many people do. Stop this killing habit! Take the salt shaker off the table. Try eating your food without added salt. Remember, any prepared food already contains too much salt. Meat contains salt, vegetables contain salt. At the present time, your taste receptors are accustomed to high salt stimulation. For this reason, as you reduce your salt intake, some foods may taste a little different, perhaps bland. This will last only a short period of time. Your taste will readjust and then you will notice that overdoses of salt are very distasteful.

Reducing your salt intake may seem like a small, insignificant step in your climb up the ladder of wellness. Not so. It can be one of the most significant. By reducing salt intake, you play an active role in minimizing your risk for high blood pressure, a stroke or a heart attack. By taking these small steps one at a time, you arrive at the top of the ladder—high-level wellness—feeling better and living longer.

CAFFEINE

Caffeine is a drug. It is probably the most overused drug in the world. Caffeine has been studied extensively. We know a great deal about it—what it does to the body and how. The overwhelming majority of coffee, tea, and cola drinkers have no idea of the action of all the caffeine they consume each day.

It is difficult to estimate the exact amount of caffeine in your brewed drinks because the product used, amount of water, and time brewed all determine caffeine concentration. The prime factor in determining caffeine content is length of brewing or steeping time. The following figures will give you a general idea of the amount of caffeine you ingest each time you have a cup or a glassful.

Caffeine Content of Various Foods

	CAFFEINE CONTENT (MILLIGRAMS/7-OUNCE SERVING)
Coffee (brewed or instant)	115–168
Decaffeinated coffee	2–9
Leaf Tea	42–94
Bagged Tea	58–140
Instant Tea	42–84
Cocoa	42–70
Cola drinks	21–56
Chocolate Bar (small)	20–35

Caffeine is a member of a group of drugs called the xanthines. Tea contains another xanthine drug called theophylline. Cocoa contains theobromine. These drugs have well-defined pharmacologic action and are prescribed today by many physicians as bronchodilator drugs. I mention this because the total drug effect from caffeine and theophylline and/or theobromine found in tea and cocoa may be greater than that found in coffee.

The action on the vital organs and body systems of the xanthines is well understood. The xanthines produce the following effects:

- stimulation of the cerebral cortex
- stimulation of the central nervous system
- stimulation of the heart muscle
- stimulation of the kidneys
- vasoconstriction
- increase in gastric secretion
- bronchodilation

The pharmocologic action of the xanthines explains why caffeine-containing products cause a mental "pick up," overall body stimulation, increased heart rate, increase in blood pressure, increase in urination, and increase in appetite.

Below is an illustration of a portion of the many actions caffeine has on various vital organs and body systems.

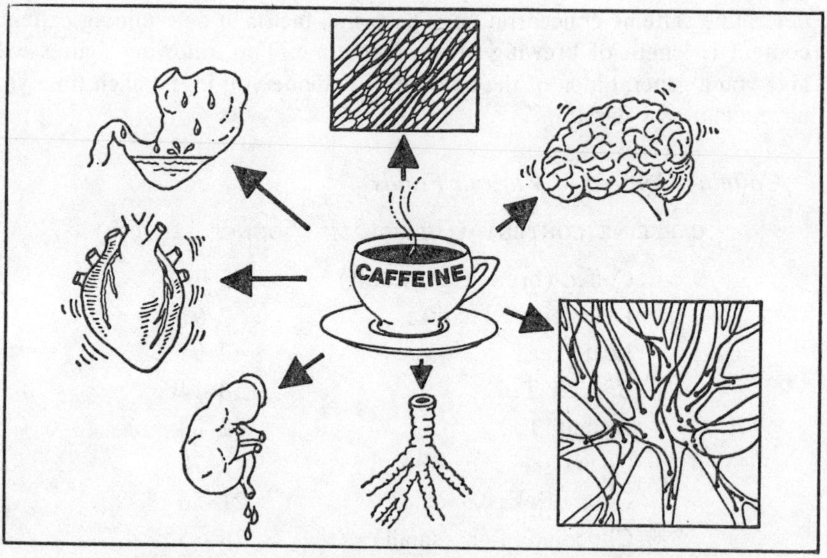

Some parts of the body affected by caffeine.

It is important for you to understand these actions.

Caffeine in moderation—one or two cups of coffee or tea per day—is probably not harmful. My concern is when consumption becomes excessive. I am referring to more than two cups per day. Then the overall body stimulation can become chronic anxiety, accelerated heart rate (harmful for the cardiac-prone individual), increased blood pressure (serious for the mildly hypertensive person), and increased gastric secretion (an ulcer for the ulcer-prone).

My intention is not to suggest that you totally eliminate these items from your diet. What I want you to do is become informed. Know that xanthine drugs exist and are present in your favorite drink or sweet. Become familiar with their pharmacological action and the symptoms they produce. Then, if you have any of these symptoms, consider the possibility that because of lack of information and knowledge you may be your own worst enemy.

If you are nervous and anxious, if you have stomach pains or gastric irritation, if your blood pressure is above normal, if you notice your heart rate is fast, if you can't sleep well, if you have any of these symptoms—stop and take a personal inventory. How many cups of coffee or tea do you drink each day? How many colas? If it's excessive, you may have the cure in front of you—reduction or elimination of the xanthine-containing products from your diet.

Often we have a tendency to equate caffeine only with coffee. Don't forget cola drinks. When referring to colas, I am not speaking of just the dark colas. Some so-called "light colas" also have caffeine. One way for you to find out is to look carefully at the label. Read and see if your favorite contains this drug. In 1974, we averaged 430 eight-ounce colas per person. Depending upon the brand, this could be an annual caffeine consumption of 8,750 to 24,080 milligrams per year. If you have any of the symptoms related to caffeine, you now know the reason.

Millions of people are inflicting preventable problems on themselves by the excessive consumption of coffee, tea, colas, cocoa, or chocolate. If you are one of them, you must exercise the self-responsibility necessary in order to alter your diet so these items are no longer consumed, or are used in moderation.

NEW WAYS OF THINKING ABOUT DIET

At the beginning of this book, it was pointed out that you would be introduced to new and different ways of thinking. Nowhere is this more evident than in eliminating poor nutrition as a negative lifestyle.

I want to introduce you to a new way to think about the word "diet." Traditionally we have defined "diet" as an alteration in eating patterns so as to lose weight. For most people, going on a "diet" means a reduction in calorie intake. This concept of determining the diet based upon caloric content alone must change.

Let me point out why. Not long ago, I was looking through a popular ladies' magazine. There was an article on how to slim down and shape up. I thought the section on exercise was excellent. The recommended diet was stated to be low in calories, which would accomplish the desired weight loss. Heading the list of recommended foods were hard-boiled eggs, shrimp, and avocados. There is no question that these foods are low in calories, but they are the highest we know of in fat and cholesterol content! The author of this diet is still under the impression that "diet" refers only to weight loss.

Starting today, I want you to change your concept of the term "diet." From now on, "diet" will mean much more than just losing or maintaining a certain body weight. Your diet, which is your master plan for high-level wellness through nutrition, will consider not only calorie consumption, but also:

- fat consumption
- cholesterol consumption
- carbohydrate consumption
- protein consumption
- salt consumption
- fiber consumption
- caffeine consumption

You must develop nutritional curiosity. Be your own detective. Start asking yourself questions like these: Is this meal high in cholesterol and fat? How much salt is in this can of soup? Does this meal provide sufficient fiber? How much simple carbohydrate versus complex carbohydrate is in my diet today? When I combine soft drinks, tea, and coffee, am I consuming too much caffeine? How much salt and fat are in that bowl of potato chips I just ate? How much simple carbohydrate is in the Super Sweet Puffies I eat for breakfast? Your "diet" must take into consideration all of these factors in addition to calories.

Sound like a pain? Perhaps so at first. But you will be surprised how easy it will become for you to automatically start monitoring your diet for more than just calories. You have the information required to raise questions. You are in the position to go on your lifelong diet, which considers the entire nutritional spectrum. Now you are beginning to think like a person who is on the way to high-level nutritional wellness—on the way to maximum longevity and high-quality life.

What's Left to Eat?

Whether I am discussing nutrition and high-level wellness with a single person or before an audience of a thousand, eventually the reaction is always the same. "What you say is fine and makes sense, but what's left to eat?" This is a good question, because it does seem that we have shot the cannon of criticism at just about all food and drink. Making the changes in your diet will be made easy by the seven-step plan you will learn about, but what would a typical daily diet look like if a person closely follows the plan?

In order to answer this question, I would like to describe for you a typical day's diet for me.

Breakfast

fruit juice (unsweetened)
fresh fruit (pineapple, grapefruit, melon, etc.)
cereal (bran type or Grape-Nuts w/wheat germ, skim milk, and fruit)
muffins (homemade, bran-based)

This breakfast is filling. Usually the muffins are left off. Cholesterol and fat are low. Complex carbohydrates and fiber are high. Total caloric content is very low. The main point is that you can quickly adjust to this breakfast. If you have eggs, sausage, buttered toast with jelly, and coffee out of habit, it may take a little determination to make the switch, but within one week you will find the above breakfast just as satisfying.

The hunger pangs of the midmorning or afternoon snack are caused out of habit. After all, you just finished breakfast or lunch several hours ago. Your digestive system has become accustomed to the midmorning and afternoon feedings and, therefore, if it is eliminated, it's unbearable. Want to know something? It's very temporary. If you can survive without these snacks for three days, the hunger pangs diminish. At the end of one week, you can go from breakfast to lunch or lunch to dinner with no problem.

If you don't want to eliminate this midmorning or midafternoon ritual, let me suggest you partake as I do on occasion:

fruit juice (grapefruit is especially good)
fresh fruit (banana, orange, apple)

This provides the complex carbohydrates needed to provide a slow release of glucose into the blood.

Lunch

I think I am personally familiar with at least 50 percent of the salad bars in the United States. Almost always I will have a medium-sized tossed salad for lunch. It is interesting to notice how many of the fast food (hamburger, fish, taco) establishments have installed self-service salad bars.

The salad for lunch is low in fat and cholesterol, high in fiber, and medium in complex carbohydrates and protein. Be careful about salad dressings. They usually are high in fats, cholesterol, and salt. A little salad dressing will go a long way, so use one spoonful—not three or four or more. Stay away from the artificial bacon chips.

Dinner

Generally I will have chicken (baked/no skin) or fish (broiled) along with vegetables. Plain baked potato or brown rice and green or yellow vegetables are excellent. A small tossed salad may be included along with dark bread. This meal provides more than enough good protein and complex carbohydrates. There are some fat and cholesterol involved, but only in small amounts.

All of these meals are without salt being added. It will take a few days to break the habit of reaching for the salt shaker before you taste the food, but soon you will be enjoying food more with only the natural salt or salt used in preparation.

You can see that my dietary recommendation to you is not to give you a long list of do's and don'ts. I am not going to say cut out all fats or all simple carbohydrates. What I want you to do is practice nutritional moderation and modification based upon the following.

Below is a short list of foods and drinks. It is my "no-no" list. I try hard to avoid these foods and drinks. Of course, I am not completely successful, but by using my mental facilities to try elimination, I actually accomplish a major reduction in intake.

Foods to Be Avoided

eggs
sausage
bacon
red meat (okay occasionally)
cheese
shellfish
canned soups, stews, spaghetti, etc.
processed meats (canned, hot dogs, cold cuts)
whole milk
ice cream
soft drinks
coffee or tea
pickles, olives, etc.
salted snacks (nuts, potato chips, pretzels, etc.)
all deep-fried foods
sugar and salt
candy and pastries and all desserts

If you can adhere to this list as I have learned to do, you will drastically reduce your intake of fat, cholesterol, simple carbohydrates, salt, and caffeine. This list of seventeen items can provide you with a giant step toward your goal of high-level nutritional wellness.

To offset the items I have eliminated from my diet, I have developed another list of foods and beverages of which I am now eating more.

Foods to Emphasize

bran muffins—homemade
bread—dark, whole grain
cereals—bran and whole grain
fish—broiled or baked
fresh fruits:
apples
bananas
berries
citrus
melon
pears
pineapple

fruit juices—all kinds
milk—skim
poultry—chicken and turkey (no skin, baked)
salads—tossed
vegetables:
all green kinds
all yellow kinds
beans—all kinds
potato—baked, plain
rice—brown

You will find this shift in diet will be easier than you think. At the end of this chapter, you will find a more comprehensive list of foods and beverages to be avoided and eaten. You are also provided with the reasons why.

I am often asked if the shifts in the diet recommended here are safe. Many will say, "I have been on a diet high in fat, cholesterol, salt, sugar, and simple sugar for many years. How can I be assured that a shift away from these foods is healthy?" This is a good question and one that requires attention. To provide an answer, I would like you to think about the following example.

The Tarahumara Indian

The nutritional habits of numerous, isolated societies have been studied. One of these groups is the Tarahumara Indian of the Sierra Madre mountains of northern Mexico. There are approximately forty thousand members of this group who have been living in this area for hundreds of years.

The Tarahumaras have been studied extensively because of their extraordinary ability in feats of physical endurance, particularly running. They have been known to run 500 miles in five days. Continuous runs of 150 to 200 miles are not unusual. The national pastime is a game called *rarahipa*. The game is not only a pastime, but also an opportunity for serious gambling. They will bet livestock, blankets, and other belongings of a substantial nature. The game is played by both men and women. In the men's game, the object is to run over mountainous terrain, kicking a hard wooden ball about four inches in diameter. The runners wear loose-fitting handmade sandals and compete against each other. They must keep the ball in front of themselves at all times. Sound difficult? The race is run at night with no lights, over a rough, mountainous course *sixty to one hundred miles long*. The women run exactly the same race, except that the course is shorter—*fifty miles*.

The Tarahumaras are medium in height, always wiry and lean. Their diet is composed almost entirely of beans and corn (complex carbohydrates and high fiber). They eat meat only several times a year. Organized medicine has been following and studying this group for years. Cardiovascular diseases are rare. Extensive blood studies are done constantly. As a group, they have one of the best HDL-LDL ratios ever recorded. Their cholesterol, triglyceride, and blood pressure are normal or below normal. Diabetes has not been seen.

This small group of Northern Hemisphere natives, who have existed for hundreds of years with little influence from the outside world, is often used as an example to prove that a simple diet can result in a body that will accomplish almost unbelievable physical feats and life-span. Studying these Indians has also proved that a diet of low or no fat is a way to minimize cardiovascular diseases.

While you probably won't be able to duplicate the accomplishments of the Tarahumaras, by starting your program for regular, sustained exercise and modifying your diet, you can add years to your life and feel better than you ever thought possible. It's all a part of the high-level wellness you are reaching for.

HOW TO ACHIEVE HIGH-LEVEL NUTRITIONAL WELLNESS

For centuries, people have been concerned and thinking about nutrition and their diet. Hippocrates, the father of modern-day medicine, said almost three thousand years ago, "Let thy food be thy medicine."

Thomas Jefferson, who lived to be eighty-four, when the life expectancy was about half that, was asked many times what it was to which he owed his longevity. His answer was always the same. He said, "You should eat breakfast like a king, lunch like a prince, and supper like a pauper."

Many people who are truly interested in beginning a life of new nutritional habits fail because they ignore the thought process. *The secret to making the required changes in your diet is not in your stomach but in your mind.* Your mind must be saturated with the facts behind how and why your present diet is destroying your vital organs and body systems. Then you must employ your program of visualization so that new signals will be sent from your mind to your body. These new signals will instruct the body that certain foods are harmful and, therefore, unacceptable. When you reach this point in nutritional wellness development, you will have no problem in eliminating those foods and drinks that are not nutritionally good. You will totally lose your appetite for them.

Now you start on the road to the highest level of nutritional wellness and will be doing everything possible to prolong your life.

Step One: *Make your personal commitment to change your eating habits and consume the most nutritious diet possible.* You have already decided that diet alteration is your number one goal. For now, you must forget about all your other negative lifestyles. Your total and undivided attention must be devoted to consuming a safer and more nutritious diet.

Your current diet is robbing you of precious years. For this reason modifying the kinds of foods and beverages you consume must become the single most important activity in your life.

I want you to write your personal commitment to high-level wellness nutrition. Your written commitment can be as short or as long as you like. It should state *how* important it is to you and *why* it is important. Write down what you plan to do in order to achieve your goal of nutritional excellence.

This written exercise is essential. By so doing you are giving your mind a command. The mind will quickly realize that you are serious about this project. In addition, the written command causes the mind to become more receptive to the information that you are going to provide. This is how you start your program to change your body regulators. They are currently set to accept foods and beverages that are unhealthy. Your committed and conditioned mind is now ready for the changes to begin.

Step Two: *Study and review again all the material and data in this chapter.* You must become your own personal expert on how and why poor nutrition destroys your vital organs and body systems and which foods are good or bad for you and why.

Know how the excessive ingestion of fats can cause red blood cells and platelet sludging and how this slows circulation. Know the role of fats in atherosclerosis, and realize that fats contain over twice the amount of calories per ounce as proteins or carbohydrates. Become familiar with foods high and low in fats. Learn about how cholesterol causes atherosclerosis. Become familiar with high-cholesterol foods. Know the difference between LDL and HDL, what they do and what influences their rise and fall have on blood cholesterol. Know the role of proteins in body function and foods that are high in proteins. Know the difference between animal and plant protein. Understand the difference between the simple and complex carbohydrates and foods high in each. Learn about the value of high-fiber content in the diet and the foods that are high in fiber. Understand how salt contributes to hypertension. Know what normal blood pressure is and what foods are naturally high in salt. Understand that caffeine is a drug and know the pharmacologic reactions it causes. Become familiar with the symptoms caused by caffeine overdosage.

Comprehend the new way of thinking about "diet." Know that your diet must include factors other than calories. Become very familiar with the foods you are going to eliminate or reduce on your new diet and those to be emphasized.

Be sure you know how and why poor nutrition is a major contributing factor to premature death—how it places a prohibition on high-level wellness and high-quality life.

At the end of this chapter you will find a formula that teaches you how to calculate the number of grams of complex carbohydrates, protein, and fat you should have each day. You will also find a list of typical foods along with fat content. From this you can see that it's easy to consume your entire allocation of fat in a single meal or a *single dish.* You are also provided with an expanded list of foods and beverages to avoid or to emphasize and the reasons why.

Step Three: *Develop the ability to mentally visualize how poor nutrition destroys your vital organs and body systems.* Study the illustrations closely. Picture in your mind how a meal high in fat causes your platelets and red blood cells to become coated with a thin layer of fat and clump together. Picture how this sludging can reduce blood flow at the capillary level. Visualize how this results in brain and body anoxia (lack of oxygen). Picture your elevated blood cholesterol causing atherosclerosis and slowing down blood flow. Develop your own mental interpretation of LDL distributing cholesterol throughout your circulatory system. Picture how the salt you eat attracts and holds water in your extracellular space, causing an increase in blood pressure and edema. Play on your mental television the program of how simple carbohydrates dump rapid and erratic amounts of glucose into the blood and how complex carbohydrates cause a smooth and constant release. Be able to vividly picture in your mind every adverse effect on your body caused by poor nutrition.

As you start to change your eating habits, you must visualize all the adverse effects reversing themselves. Picture the formed elements of the blood no longer fat-coated and sticky. Visualize maximum blood flow at the capillary level, and brain and body receiving maximum oxygen. Picture your HDL increasing and picking up more cholesterol and carrying it to the liver. Think of your atherosclerosis as disappearing and your arteries clean and elastic. Be able to mentally visualize each of the individual harmful effects of poor nutrition reversed as your diet changes.

Step Four: *Write a summary of everything you learn about how and why poor nutrition destroys vital organs and body systems.* You will learn quickly if you take notes while you are studying the material in this chapter. You will also retain the material longer. Review all of the specific actions of poor nutrition on your body which you are going to visualize. For example, how cholesterol causes atherosclerosis, the differences between how simple and complex carbohydrates release glucose into the blood, or how salt aggravates hypertension. Now, write a detailed summary of everything you have learned.

Include in your written summary all the foods and drinks you want to reduce or eliminate from your diet and those you want to increase.

You should feel free to experiment in the creation of your own visualization illustrations. As you write your summary of all the harmful effects, transpose them into your own drawings. Don't be concerned about how accurate your illustrations are. The main point is for you to become involved in establishing in your mind the "before and after" pictures of the effects of poor and proper nutrition. Illustrations which you create will be very meaningful to you.

Step Five: *Practice your visualization program every morning upon waking, at lunch, dinner, bedtime, and any time you are tempted to consume food or drink that will result in poor nutrition.* After you have perfected your ability to visualize your nutritional program, it is essential that you have a fixed schedule. This schedule will be invaluable in getting you into the habit of visualizing your way to high-level nutritional wellness.

You must start each day, as soon as you wake, with your program. While still in bed, run through your mind the pictures of how and why poor nutrition is destroying your vital organs and body systems. Picture how too much fat causes your red blood cells to stick together. How a low-fiber diet is harmful. How excessive salt can cause hypertension. Then picture what will happen as everything returns to normal under the influence of your new nutritional program. Non-sticky red blood cells and platelets, clean and elastic arteries, high ratio of HDL, the proper amount of water attracting sodium, etc.

Other times for visualization should initially be associated with your accustomed routine, such as midmorning and afternoon break, lunch, and dinner. Visualization is a new mental exercise, and a part of mental fitness. It requires discipline on your part as you begin, but it will become habit in a short period of time.

All visualization practice is good, but the best time is at night just before going to sleep. Your mind functions and can be conditioned during sleep. Before going to sleep, replay your entire visualization program from beginning to end—what your body systems and vital organs now look like as a result of poor nutrition and what they are going to look like after the readjustment in your diet.

We live in a world of nutritional temptation. All of us are subject to these temptations. When you find yourself in these situations, visualize. You will be amazed how quickly visualization will totally remove the momentary desire for food or drink not in your diet.

Step Six: *Determine and write down a schedule or target date when poor nutrition will no longer be a part of your life.* If you are like most people, you will be involved in a number of corrections that must be made in your diet. For this reason, you should have a predetermined written goal. This goal will be that point in time when your fat, cholesterol, protein, carbohydrate, salt, and fiber intake will be where you want them.

The mind always responds best if it has a clearly defined goal to shoot for. Part of this goal is a time schedule whereby you will accomplish your goal.

Step Seven: *Develop a vivid mental picture of you without poor nutrition as a part of your life.* This is one of the most important parts of your visualization programs. You must give your mind the ultimate goal you are striving to achieve. This goal is *you* in the highest state of nutritional wellness. In addition to visualizing all vital organs and body systems at the highest level of wellness, you must also visualize yourself actually consuming your new diet, which takes into consideration not only calories, but also fats, cholesterol, protein, simple and complex carbohydrates, fiber, and salt. Picture yourself becoming what you eat and eating what is best for you.

You now have at your disposal a program that will allow you to beam with personal pride and nutritional wellness. Poor nutrition is one of the most devastating of all negative lifestyles. And it's completely unnecessary. You can eat all the *right* foods and have a fabulous diet. Apply this program now and you will be like the many others who have learned HOW TO EAT, DRINK, AND BE HEALTHY.

ADDITIONAL HELPFUL HINTS

At the end of each chapter you are provided with a brief outline of practical information, tips, and hints that are intended to supplement your visualization program. When used in conjunction with visualization, they will help you eliminate your negative lifestyle.

These practical hints to help you in achieving a more nutritious diet show you how to calculate the number of grams of carbohydrates, protein, and fat you should eat daily. You are also provided with a brief list of foods to be avoided or to be emphasized.

Many foods have on the label information about the number of calories and grams of carbohydrates, protein, and fat per serving. In order to make this information meaningful, you must know how much of these four components you should have each day. There is a simple formula you can use.

A male who does light work, is twenty-three to fifty years old, stands 5 feet 11 inches tall and weighs 156 pounds needs about 2,700 calories daily. A female of the same age doing similar work, who is 5 feet 4 inches tall and weighs 126 pounds requires about 2,000 calories each day.

Your daily caloric intake should come from the following:

complex carbohydrates	60 percent
protein	20 percent
fat	20 percent

These figures could be plus or minus 5 percent.

In order to determine the number of grams of complex carbohydrates, protein, and fat you should consume each day, do the following:

Multiply the percent of complex carbohydrates by the total daily caloric intake (60% × 2,700 = 1,620). Thus, for the male 1,620 calories should be in complex carbohydrates.

There are 4 calories per gram of complex carbohydrates and protein. Therefore, divide 4 into 1,620 (1,620 ÷ 4 = 405). The male requires *405 grams of complex carbohydrates daily.*

To find the grams of protein use the same formula except multiply by 20% (2,700 × 20% = 540) (540 ÷ 4 = 135). The male needs *135 grams of protein each day.*

There are 9 calories per gram of fat so the division is by 9 instead of 4. Multiply 2,700 by 20% (2,700 × 20% = 540). Divide 540 by 9 (540 ÷ 9 = 60). The male should have *60 grams of fat daily.*

Using this same formula, you will find that each day, the *female* should consume *300 grams of complex carbohydrates, 100 grams of protein,* and *44 grams of fat.*

Since special attention to daily fat intake is essential to high-level wellness, you must become familiar with the fat content of the foods and beverages you consume. Below is an abbreviated list of popular foods and beverages along with the grams of fat per average serving.

Average Fat Content of Various Foods

FOOD OR BEVERAGE	SERVING	AMOUNT OF FAT
Biscuits—canned	2 small	10 grams
Butter	1 tbs	11 grams
Cheese—cream	1 oz	10 grams
Cheese—cheddar	1 oz	9 grams
Cheese—cottage	½ cup	5 grams
Chili—canned	3 oz	15 grams
Chips—potato	1 oz	11 grams
Corned beef hash—canned	3 oz	13 grams
Hamburger	3 oz	17 grams
Hot dog	one	12 grams
Ice cream	½ cup	10 grams
Lamb chop with fat	3 oz	33 grams
Margarine	1 tbs	11 grams
Mayonnaise	1 tbs	11 grams
Milk—whole	1 cup	9 grams
Oils—corn, peanut, vegetable, safflower	1 tbs	14 grams
Peanut butter	2 tbs	17 grams
Pork chop with fat	3 oz	21 grams
Potpie—beef	4½″ diameter	33 grams
Sausage—link	2 links	11 grams
Steak sirloin with fat	3 oz	27 grams
Tostada	1 oz	7 grams
Tuna in oil	3 oz	14 grams

After looking at this list, you can see why it's easy for the *male* to consume more than *60 grams of fat* daily and for the *female* to go over *44 grams.* Calculate the maximum number of grams of fat you should have each day. Then, from the information on the package, become aware of how much fat you eat daily.

Following is a list of foods and beverages which high-level wellness forbids. The reasons why are listed. Next, is another list that presents you with what you should emphasize. Again, the reasons are provided.

Foods and Beverages to Avoid

PRODUCT	WHY?
Animal fat	very high in saturated fat
Avocados	high in fat
Bacon, ham, pork	very high in fat and salt
Beef stew—canned	high in fat and salt
Biscuits—commercial mix	high in fat and salt
Bouillon	very high in salt
Bread—white	dark is more nutritious
Cakes, cookies, pastries	high in simple carbohydrates and fat
Candy—all kinds	very high in simple carbohydrates
Cereal—sugar-coated	very high in simple carbohydrates
Cheese—all kinds	high in fat and salt
Chili—canned	high in fat and salt
Chips—potato, corn, tortilla	very high in fat and salt
Chocolate in any form	high in caffeine
Coconut	high in fat
Coffee	very high in caffeine
Corned beef or pastrami	high in fat and salt
Crackers—salted	high in salt
Cream—including nondairy	high in fat
Deep-fried foods of all kinds	very high in fat
Duck and goose	high in fat
Eggs and products containing eggs	very high in cholesterol
French toast	high in cholesterol
Frozen dinners and dishes	high in salt and fat
Gravy—mixes and cream sauce	high in salt and fat
Ice cream	high in fat
Jelly and jam	very high in simple carbohydrates
Luncheon meats—cold cuts, hot dogs, bologna, salami	very high in salt and fat
Mayonnaise	high in cholesterol and salt
Margarine	high in fat

PRODUCT	WHY?
Meat—red	high in fat and cholesterol
Meat—canned	high in fat and salt
Meat—organ—liver, kidney, brain, sweetbreads	very high in cholesterol
Milk—whole	high in fat
Muffins—commercial mix	high in fat, salt, and simple carbohydrates
Nuts—all kinds	high in fat
Oils—corn, cottonseed, olive, peanut, safflower, soybean	high in fat
Olives	very high in salt
Pancakes, waffles with syrup	high in simple carbohydrates and fat
Peanut butter	high in salt and fat
Pies	high in simple carbohydrates and fat
Pickles	very high in salt
Pizza	high in fat and salt
Pretzels	high in salt
Salad dressing	high in fat and salt
Shellfish—shrimp, oysters, clams, lobster, crabs	high in cholesterol
Soft drinks	usually very high in simple carbohydrates and caffeine
Soups—canned or dry mix	very high in salt and fat
Spaghetti—canned or mix	high in salt
Tuna—in oil	high in fat
Tea	high in caffeine

Foods and Beverages to Emphasize

BEVERAGES	
milk—skim	low in fat, high in protein
juices orange grapefruit grape cranberry tomato—low sodium	high in complex carbohydrates
decaffeinated coffee	low in caffeine
decaffeinated tea	low in caffeine
POULTRY	
chicken, turkey (no skin—baked)	low in fat, high in protein

FISH	
all kinds (broiled)	low in fat, high in protein
FRUITS	
apples pears plums apricots oranges grapefruit tangerines berries cherries pineapple bananas melons grapes peaches watermelon	all listed fruits are high in complex carbohydrates, very low in fat and cholesterol, low in salt, high in fiber, and low in calories
VEGETABLES	
potatoes rice beans lima navy pinto kidney carrots cabbage asparagus beets broccoli Brussels sprouts cauliflower corn lettuce tomatoes	all listed vegetables are high in complex carbohydrates, very low in fat and cholesterol, low in salt, high in fiber, and low in calories; the legumes (beans) are moderately high in protein
BREAD	
dark, whole grain muffins—bran base	high in complex carbohydrates, low in calories, high in fiber

CEREALS	
bran type oatmeal—not instant shredded wheat raw wheat germ	very high in fiber, low in fat and cholesterol, low in calories, high in complex carbohydrates
SNACKS	
all fresh fruits raw vegetables carrots cabbage cauliflower broccoli bran muffin dry dark toast cold chicken cold turkey fruit juices	very low in calories, low in fat and cholesterol, low in salt, high in fiber, chicken and turkey high in protein

7. HOW TO GET YOUR WEIGHT DOWN STARTING NOW!

"The longer the belt, the shorter the life."

As this is being written, I am sitting in a comfortable chaise lounge at water's edge on the Gulf of Mexico. I am at a popular resort city and the tourist business is at season's high. The beach is crowded with vacationers from throughout the southeastern part of the United States and beyond.

If you would like a firsthand visual documentary on the problem of obesity in the United States, you should be with me today. Surveying thousands of people who are in various designs of swimwear, it is easy to appreciate the fact that 40 percent of the people in this country are obese.

As I observe people walking up and down the beach, several facts become clear. For young people (fifteen to twenty-two years of age) obesity is usually not a major problem. In observing young couples—the ones with children from three to seven years old—the wife is more often obese than the husband. Studies have confirmed this. Many reasons have been advanced for this increased obesity among young housewives. Some of them are: being at home all day presents tremendous opportunities for overeating; the frustration of trying to raise a family and maintain the home leads to the desire for an outlet and often overeating becomes the compensating factor; the young husband may be moving up the corporate ladder and has less time for the wife, with more frustration for her. Gratification is gained through eating. In this age group, the husband may be slightly overweight but not as much as the wife.

After age thirty-five, a change can be observed in the obesity pattern between the wife and husband. At this time the husband starts to gain weight. Numerous reasons are involved. Usually the husband has been involved in his job for ten to twelve years. Often recognition and advancement have not come as quickly as he feels they should. This results in frustration, which can be satisfied by drink and food. The husband observes the wife getting uncontrollably overweight and develops the attitude that if she doesn't care, neither does he. Many times the job itself requires a certain amount of entertainment or image-playing. Both may require considerable exposure to and consumption of alcohol and food.

One of the most serious factors involved in the husband's gaining weight during these years is lack of exercise. From the standpoint of physical fitness, the majority of men go into retirement after graduating from high school or college. As the eating pattern increases and exercise remains constant or declines, the inevitable result is weight gain.

As men and women move beyond the age of forty-five years, obesity usually becomes a more definite problem for both. At this point, obesity is probably equally distributed, with most people being overweight. There are numerous explanations for this. As people become older (I am not suggesting that over forty-five is old!) some have a tendency to become less interested in the physical aspects of the body and more interested in the pleasures provided by eating. Often regular physical exercise ceases completely. It is a known medical fact that after age forty-five the rate of metabolism slows down. These are just a few of the numerous explanations as to why people over forty-five have difficulty coping with the problems of obesity.

As I have indicated at the beginning of this book, I have personally been down the road of obesity and therefore can appreciate some of your problems. I can also speak with some degree of authority on the myths that are connected with obesity.

Since you and I have shared a common problem, I will address the situation in a frank and perhaps blunt way. No offense is intended, but if you are serious about achieving and maintaining ideal body weight, we must communicate on an honest and straightforward basis.

First, let's establish several definitions. Throughout this chapter, I refer to obesity. Technically, there is a difference between being overweight and being obese. According to the textbooks, you are overweight if your body weight is 10 to 20 percent above ideal weight. You are obese if you are more than 20 percent over ideal weight. Let's translate these into real numbers. If you are a man of average frame size and are 6 feet tall, you should weigh 159 pounds (undressed). If, in fact, you weight 175 to 191 pounds, you are overweight. If you weigh over 191 pounds, you are obese. If you are a woman of average frame size and are 5 feet 4 inches tall, you should weigh 123 pounds (undressed). If you weigh 135 to 147 pounds, you are overweight. If your weight is over 147 pounds, you are obese.

Since being overweight usually leads to obesity, the problem of overweight is just as important as obesity. For this reason, in this book no distinction will be made between overweight and obesity. The term obesity is used in referring to any condition in which the person is above ideal weight.

Now let's dispel a few archaic assumptions about obesity:

1) Obese people are *not* happier people. Often individuals who are obese put on a façade of happiness—a jolly personality—in order to cover their real dissatisfaction with themselves and the anxieties they have. Obese people are usually frustrated about their problem and in the majority of cases want to do something about it.

2) Fad diets don't work. Last Christmas, one of my sons gave me a book that condensed and commented on books that have been written on 128 different diets. They ranged from the grapefruit diet to the drinking-man's diet. These diets don't work for several reasons. In many instances, they are not practical. One cannot live forever on a diet of grapefruit, rice, or alcohol. Second, fad diets usually do nothing to change basic eating patterns. You are obese because the relationship between your hunger signals and the body's real need for nourishment have gotten out of adjustment. Your hunger signals are going off too often and, in addition, you eat when you are not truly hungry.

3) It is estimated that less than 5 percent of those who are obese have glandular or other physical problems. Thus, the person who tries to rationalize obesity with the idea that something organic is causing the problem is usually looking for an easy way out.

4) Taking pills is never a long-term solution to your problem. There is no question that certain drugs can and will reduce the appetite. Thus you will lose weight. However, numerous studies point out that after the pills are stopped, old eating habits return and lost weight is quickly regained. In addition, certain kinds of appetite-suppressant pills can cause dangerous side effects.

   Diet supplements are similar. You will lose weight while using them, but one cannot live for a lifetime on diet supplements.

> Weight is regained because there is no permanent change made in eating habits. Unless you change your eating habits, there is no long-term weight loss.

I trust that I have not been too harsh, but it is important for you to understand from the beginning that you have a problem that is a negative lifestyle, not unlike the others discussed in this book. Obesity, smoking, excessive consumption of alcohol, poor nutrition, inability to cope with everyday stress, and lack of regular exercise are all kissing cousins. They are the results of *acquired or learned* habits or behavioral patterns. It is important for you to understand this, because any acquired habit can be changed. You are now on your way to learning how.

In this chapter, when the reference is made to "food," it is intended to mean food and drink. With few exceptions, all foods and drinks (or solids and liquids) contain calories. Thus, the reference to food means caloric consumption from both solids and liquids. Likewise, the reference to eating refers to both eating and drinking.

Americans have a love affair with eating. A recent half-page article in the New York *Post* was headlined: SEX OUTVOTED, FOOD WINS. The newspaper was featuring excerpts from the just-published *Book of Lists No. 2*. It pointed out that in an ABC-Harris Survey, 1,442 adults were interviewed across the United States. Each participant was read the following statement by the interviewer: "I'm going to read you a list of things other people say they do with their leisure time. As I read each one, tell me whether you do it frequently, occasionally, or not at all." Here are the things adults say they do most frequently with their leisure time:

MEN

RANK		
1	Eating	54%
2	Watching television	41%
3	Fixing things around the house	41%
4	Listening to the radio	39%
5	Listening to music at home	35%
6	Reading books	30%
7	Outdoor activities/hiking, fishing, boating	30%
8	Having sex	29%
9	Social activities/dining out, dancing, parties	25%
10	Participating in sports like golf, tennis, swimming	23%
11	Hobbies/photography, woodwork, etc.	22%
12	Trying to earn extra money	19%
13	Taking naps	17%
14	Participating in church or club activities	17%
15	Just getting away for a change of scenery	17%

WOMEN

RANK		
1	Eating	54%
2	Reading books	47%
3	Listening to music at home	42%
4	Watching television	40%
5	Listening to the radio	40%
6	Fixing things around the house	31%
7	Participating in church or club activities	28%
8	Social activities/dining out, dancing, parties	25%
9	Having sex	22%
10	Hobbies/photography, woodwork, etc.	19%
11	Participating in sports like golf, tennis, swimming	15%
12	Trying to earn extra money	15%
13	Continuing your education	15%
14	Just getting away for a change of scenery	14%
15	Outdoor activities/hiking, fishing, boating	13%

It is astounding to realize that, based on this representative sample, eating is America's most frequent and favorite pastime.

While this may be surprising, think for a moment. When something really special happens or when you have an occasion to celebrate, how do you recognize the occasion? If you are like 80 percent of the population, you go out to eat! When friends drop in, the most frequent reaction is to offer them food or drink. Many find it difficult or impossible to watch television, go to a movie or a ball game without eating and drinking. The midmorning and midafternoon office breaks, which were intended to provide a period of relaxation, have turned into minimeals for the majority.

The main point is that in the United States eating has become an obsession for many people. In fact, for some, eating is the "Magnificent Obsession." Eating has become a ritual to which many are attracted and participate—hungry or not.

FACTORS THAT CAUSE YOU TO OVEREAT

Why have we as a nation become so obsessed with eating? Why has eating become the number one social event in the United States? Why has eating become our most important form of entertainment? Why is it that on numerous occasions we eat when not really hungry? Dozens of potential answers have been expounded in an effort to explain our almost fanatical interest in eating. As you start on your program for permanent weight reduction, it would be important for us to briefly review a few of the many proposed reasons. They are not presented in any order of importance.

Eating fills a basic psychological need. Everyone has certain basic psychological needs. These may be the need to love and be loved, the need to contribute, the need to be wanted, the need for acceptance, the need for recognition, the need for communication, etc. In all or many cases, the individual finds these needs cannot be fulfilled. When this occurs, a substitute is required to satisfy these needs. Eating is always an easy substitute.

Lack of security and rejection are other psychological reasons for excessive eating. When a person feels unwanted or insecure, one unconscious way to satisfy the mind and body is through eating.

Psychological needs that are impossible to achieve or realize are replaced by eating. Eating, which to a great degree was intended as a means to an end, to sustain body function, has become for many a psychological pacifier.

Early habits. For some incorrect and unexplained reason, we have always felt that a fat baby is a healthy baby. If you are a parent, how often have you instructed, coerced, or punished your children into "cleaning the plate"? How often have you admonished the family to eat everything (whether hungry or not) so that food will not be wasted? The point is that in many cases (I am not aware of any hard data on the exact percentage) parents routinely *force* infants and small children to eat. The basic instinct of hunger doesn't matter. The young person should eat copious meals in order to make mother happy. Many future problems with obesity are started very early in life as excessive eating habits are established by an overzealous parent.

Availability. In this day and age, we are virtually swimming in a sea of food and drink. I once read that in the United States you are usually *never* more than ten minutes away from food. This may be the refrigerator at home, the local grocery store, the vending machine at the office, the local candy store, the concession stand at numerous entertainment events, etc. The plethora of food that surrounds us at all times makes it extremely easy to eat based upon availability instead of hunger.

Advertising. It is a known fact that appetite reacts to suggestion. This suggestion can come from any of the five senses. When you smell food being cooked, imagine a favorite tasty dish, or see one of your favorite foods, what happens? The gastric juices start to flow, the hunger pangs start, and you become hungry. The food industry is one of the most clever in the country. They know the impact high-quality advertising can have on increasing the sale of their products. Did you ever study the advertisements in any of the popular ladies' magazines? If you are not hungry when you pick up the magazine, I can assure you your appetite will be stimulated before you put it down. Television advertisements for food and drink have the same impact.

Numerous experiments have been done with subliminal food and drink advertising in the movies and television. The product is flashed on the screen for a fraction of a second. It is almost as if you are not sure you really saw it. Even though the eye may not recognize the product being shown, the mind will. Let's say the subliminal advertising is for a particular soft drink and popcorn. The immediate sale of these products always goes up significantly.

I do not want to give the impression that I am against food advertising. Everyone has the right to advertise their products. No one does it more effectively than the food industry. What you must keep in mind is that if you are obese and trying to lose weight, don't knowingly and actively engage in a routine study of food and drink advertising.

Types of food. During the past twenty years, we have become a "junk food" society. For many, numerous meals are taken at fast food establishments or from vending machines. We have become a nation on the run most of the time. This leads to snack-type meals. Usually meals of this type are very high in calories. Want an example? Let's say you are on a 1,500 calories per day diet and you have a cheeseburger, small french fries, and small cola for lunch. You have just ingested approximately 1,115 calories. You have consumed at lunch almost your total calorie intake for the twenty-four-hour period. Some place partial blame for our national obesity problem on how our society has changed eating habits over recent years. These changes have been to more snack-type meals, which are usually very high in calories.

There are no doubt numerous other factors that could be presented as possible explanations for why we are obsessed with eating—why obesity is a national epidemic. However, none of the previously mentioned factors reflect the real reasons for our runaway desire for eating. They may be complicating and contributing factors but not the prime reason.

WHY DO YOU OVEREAT?

Now, let's examine the real reason for your obesity. I'm not talking about the simple explanation that you are obese because you eat too much, because you ingest more calories than you use. From a physical standpoint, these explanations and observations are correct, but what you need to know is *why* you eat too much and *why* you consume more calories than you use.

Your body requires a constant amount of energy and nutritional input for normal healthy life function. This is supplied by carbohydrates, protein, fat, vitamins, and minerals. The relationship between the needs for these factors and appetite is another of the body's magnificent systems of checks and balances. The brain, through the hypothalamus, can detect body needs for nourishment. When certain nutrients drop below a given point, the fact is detected by the brain and signals are sent out that activate the appetite system and you become hungry. This is a finely tuned feedback system which, under normal conditions, will maintain a person with ideal body weight. In other words, your appetite is supposed to become activated by the mind only when there are definite body needs. In your case, the connection between the mind and body has developed a short circuit. Your appetite becomes active when there is no actual body requirement.

What went wrong? Why and how has your body-need–appetite mechanism become maladjusted? One of the basic problems with obese people is that they eat when they are not hungry and/or eat beyond the point where the appetite is satisfied. When this occurs, the normal feedback mechanism from the satisfied appetite to the mind is destroyed. It's like a fast downhill moving eighteen-wheeler without brakes. It is out of control. Because of eating from habit or because of availability of food, the regulator between the mind and body has a malfunction.

As has been pointed out, the mind can be trained and influenced. This is accomplished by providing information—the *hows* and *whys*—to the mind. In your case, the mind, because of your eating habits, has been influenced to have the "ready to eat" regulator turned on high all the time.

I assume that the majority of you reading this chapter are obese to some degree. You would like to lose weight, either a few or many pounds. Some of you have gone on numerous diets, lost weight, and gained it back. For others, this may be your first attempt to secure control of your obesity problem. Regardless of what has happened in the past, you must begin by regaining control of your body-need–appetite regulator. You must return again to a situation in which your appetite turns on only when your body needs nutritional input and turns off when the body's needs are satisfied.

The big question is: How is this accomplished? First you must realize that there can be no high-level wellness contained in a body that is obese. You must know and understand your own responsibility as it pertains to achieving and maintaining ideal body weight. The way you acquire this self-responsibility is through education. You must, today, start on a program to educate your mind as to *how* and *why* obesity is harmful to your vital organs and body systems. Due to lack of basic information, your body regulators are currently adjusted to constant overeating as an okay activity. The mind does not comprehend or understand the disastrous effects of being overweight. What you must do is saturate your mind as to exactly how and why obesity destroys vital organs and vital systems and causes premature death. Once this is accomplished, your body regulators readjust. They readjust to the setting that obesity is harmful. They readjust the appetite cycle so that you will be hungry only when there is a basic body need for nourishment. They readjust so that you will be content and happy not eating between meals, becoming filled on less food, and losing your desire for high-calorie foods.

The important fact for you to realize is that your answer to losing weight and maintaining ideal body weight forever is not in fad diets, pills, or diet supplements. These are all crutches that bend and break with the passing of time. The permanent answer to your problem is to *change your eating habits.* The only way this can be accomplished is by influencing your mind and gaining control over the signals that are transmitted. The program that I will teach you accomplishes this. You are about to launch into a program that will result in weight loss to the extent you desire, with the assurance that the weight will never be gained back again.

BODY FORMS

From the time we are very young, we are taught that "all people are created equal." After all these years, I hate to disillusion you, but it just isn't so. All people are not created equal, at least in body form. It is essential that you know and understand body forms as you begin your personal program for permanent weight reduction.

From the moment of conception, your body form is determined. In the first weeks of gestation, as the cells are being developed, your body form starts to develop.

There are three distinctly different body forms. They are illustrated on page 146:

The body form on the left is the ectomorph. The ectomorph is slightly taller than average and tends to be on the lean and wiry side. This is the individual who can eat copious amounts of food and usually not gain weight. Those of us who are not ectomorphs observe their huge eating habits and their slim bodies and with a sigh of envy say, "How can they do it? How can they eat so much and stay so slim?" The answer is: They have nothing to do with it. Their body form dictates that the ectomorph usually will not have a problem with obesity.

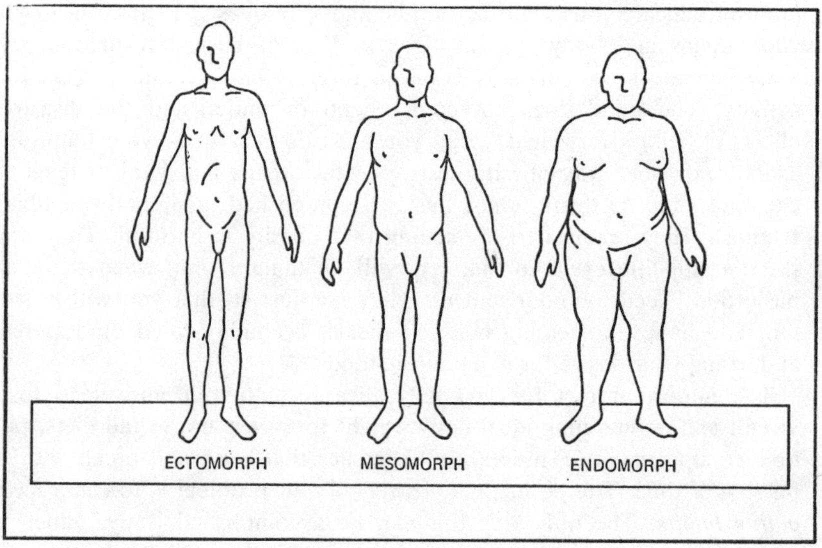

Body Forms

On the far right is the endomorph. The endomorph is shorter than average with a body disposition that can best be described as soft. By nature, the endomorph has a natural tendency to gain weight easily. Most endomorphs can walk up to a table full of food, inhale deeply, and gain weight. I have never read any clinical reports to document this observation, but every endomorph I know swears it's a fact.

In the middle is the mesomorph. The mesomorph, to a degree, is a combination of the ectomorph and endomorph. They are average height and usually somewhat muscular in body composition. In regard to weight-gaining tendencies, they fall somewhere in between the ecto- and endomorph. This body form suggests that obesity can be a problem, but with a certain amount of discipline, ideal body weight can be maintained.

I have read dozens of books on weight control and this is the first one I am aware of that recognizes that different body forms are real and do exist. It's easy to understand why individuals who are weight-control advocates want to avoid the issue. They are concerned that everyone who is obese will immediately plead that they are an endomorph and, therefore, "God intended me to be fat, so why be concerned about it?" I give you more credit than that. I want you to know that if you are an endomorph, you may have a more difficult time in achieving and maintaining normal body weight. This is not to suggest that it is impossible for the endomorph to have a trim and fit body. Identifying and knowing your body form is an

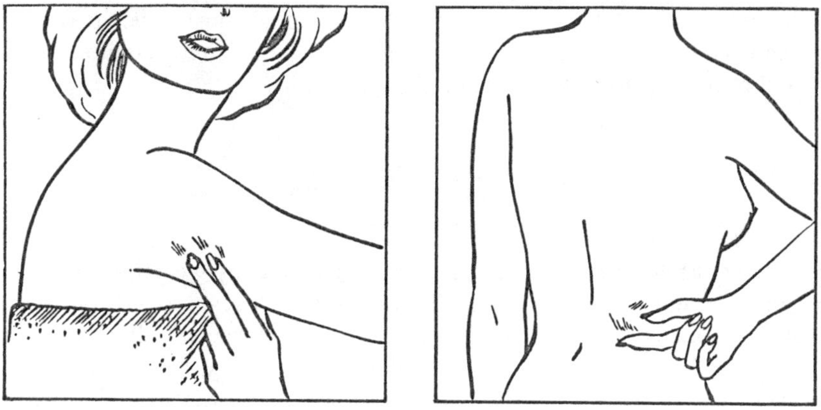

Pinch Test

weight range is considerable. For this reason, if you are on the high side, you can be within normal limits and still be obese.

Remember, the determination of your obesity or lack of it is something of which you must be aware and convinced. Obesity determination will probably be based on a combination of the previously outlined methods. For further assistance in determining if you are obese, you may make reference to the following weight chart.

Men

Height in Shoes	Weight in Pounds (in Indoor Clothing)		
(1″ HEELS)	SMALL FRAME	MEDIUM FRAME	LARGE FRAME
5′ 2″	112–120	118–129	126–141
3″	115–124	121–133	129–144
4″	118–126	124–136	132–148
5″	121–129	127–139	135–152
6″	124–133	130–143	138–156
7″	128–137	134–147	142–161
8″	132–141	138–152	147–166
9″	136–145	142–156	151–170
10″	140–150	146–160	155–174
11″	144–154	150–165	159–179
6′ 0″	148–158	154–170	164–184
1″	152–162	158–175	168–189
2″	156–167	162–180	173–194
3″	160–171	167–185	178–199
4″	164–175	172–190	182–204

important piece of information which your mind must have in (send out the proper signals and readjust your appetite regulators will result in a permanent change in eating habits.

ARE YOU OBESE?

We must address the question of what is ideal body weight and h you determine if you are obese. This question is not as easy to an it may initially seem. There are numerous formulas and charts t tell you what you should weigh and if you are obese according t ages. The problem is in different frame sizes, that is, skeletal st Some people have a frame that is larger than others. For this rea expect everyone of the same age and height to weigh the same is sonable.

When conducting Wellness Seminars, one question that comes u is, "What is obesity?" Others ask, "How can I tell if I am obese?"

Numerous methods have been developed to help you know if y overweight. Some are simple, some are very complex and compli would like to share several with you.

One way is to simply take body inventory. Get undressed and yourself closely in a full-length mirror. Look from the front, sid back. Are you pleased with what you see? Are you satisfied wit body? According to your standards, is your body attractive? Ho your body compare with the way it looked five years ago? ten yea twenty years ago? Try to view yourself as others do. Most people I rarely do this. It's another of those situations we take for granted take an obese body for granted. This self-analysis of the body is al good place to start in determining if you are obese. Take it seriou careful obesity body check is a good place to start on a program of reduction.

Another way to determine if you are overweight is the "pinch te conduct this test, grasp the tissue on the back side of the uppe Pinch it gently. Fatty tissue has a tendency to concentrate in thi When you pinch, if the tissue between your fingers is one inch o across, you are obese. The same prodecure is used in pinching the on the waistline halfway between the middle of the back and th Again, if you are able to pinch up more than one inch, you are obese.

Numerous actuary tables have been prepared which tell you, upon your height, age, and body-frame size, how much you should Charts of this type are a general guideline and require that one be pletely honest when defining frame size. Another problem is th

Women

Height in Shoes (2″ HEELS)	Weight in Pounds (in Indoor Clothing) SMALL FRAME	MEDIUM FRAME	LARGE FRAME
4′10″	92–98	96–107	104–119
11″	94–101	98–110	106–122
5′ 0″	96–104	101–113	109–125
1″	99–107	104–116	112–118
2″	102–110	107–119	115–131
3″	105–113	110–122	118–134
4″	108–116	113–126	121–138
5″	111–119	116–130	125–142
6″	114–123	120–135	129–146
7″	118–127	124–139	133–150
8″	122–131	128–143	137–154
9″	126–135	132–147	141–158
10″	130–140	136–151	145–163
11″	134–144	140–155	149–168
6′ 0″	138–148	144–159	153–173

This table is adapted from the Metropolitan Life Insurance study of overweight. (If undressed, deduct 3 pounds for men and 2 pounds for women.)

WHY DO YOU GAIN WEIGHT?

We have already considered several of the major psychological factors in overeating. These are important facts and must be a part of any program to increase the level of knowledge about losing weight. However, I want to caution you about placing too much emphasis on the psychological to the exclusion of the physical. Regardless of the reasons why, you have gained weight because your caloric intake has exceeded your caloric need.

Let's review the fundamentals of the physical side of obesity. Technically, a calorie is the amount of energy required to increase one gram of water one degree in temperature. If this sounds complicated, just remember a calorie is a measure of energy. We are constantly using energy. Twenty-four hours a day, as long as you are alive and breathing, you are using energy which can be expressed as calories. You use the least number of calories when you are sleeping. As you become increasingly involved in physical activities, the amount of energy required and the number of calories used go up. If you are standing up, you require more energy than when lying down—more when walking as compared to standing—more when running as compared to walking. The more intense the activity, the greater the amount of energy required, which results in an increase in the number of calories used.

On the other hand, you have direct control over the number of calories you eat in order to meet this energy demand. Herein lies the essence of weight control. Foods and beverages vary drastically in calorie content. You must be able to increase calorie usage and decrease the intake. In order to do this, you must have a general idea of how many calories the average person needs per day to *maintain* present body weight.

How many calories do you need each day to provide normal body energy? It depends upon several factors. Your age makes a difference. As you grow older, your metabolism slows and calorie requirements decline. Your height and weight are factors. The greater the body mass, the more calories you need to *maintain* present body weight.

The National Academy of Sciences points out in the 1980 revised *Recommended Dietary Allowances* that the following calories are what you need to provide adequate body energy and maintain present weight. If you want to lose weight, you must consume considerably less.

Males

AGE	WEIGHT	HEIGHT	CALORIES NEEDED
11–14	99 lbs	5′2″	2,700
15–18	145 lbs	5′9″	2,800
19–22	154 lbs	6′0″	2,900
23–50	154 lbs	6′0″	2,700
51–75	154 lbs	6′0″	2,400
76 +	154 lbs	6′0″	2,050

Females

AGE	WEIGHT	HEIGHT	CALORIES NEEDED
11–14	101 lbs	5′2″	2,200
15–18	120 lbs	5′4″	2,100
19–22	120 lbs	5′4″	2,100
23–50	120 lbs	5′4″	2,000
51–75	120 lbs	5′4″	1,800
76 +	120 lbs	5′4″	1,600

Taken from: *Recommended Dietary Allowances,* Ninth Revised Edition (1980), with the permission of the National Academy of Sciences, Washington, D.C.

These data are based upon a person who is involved in moderately active work or play. If you do strenuous work or jog ten miles every day, you must adjust the calories up slightly. If you are behind a desk all day with no exercise, adjust downward. Very slight adjustment should be made if you are taller or shorter, or heavier or lighter than listed.

Caloric expenditure has been carefully studied and explained. Exact studies have determined the approximate number of calories you utilize for a variety of physical activities. Some of these are listed below.

ACTIVITY	CALORIES 1 MIN.	CALORIES 10 MIN.	CALORIES 30 MIN.
sleeping	1	10	30
sitting and talking	1.25	12.5	37.5
standing	1.5	12.5	45
strolling at less than a 30-min. mile; light housework; gardening; raking	2	20	60
walking a 20-min. mile; cycling a 10-min. mile; bowling; cleaning windows; mowing grass; horseback riding	4	40	120
table tennis; fencing; volleyball; tennis-racquetball (doubles); golfing (walking); calisthenics; shoveling snow	5	50	150
walking a 15-min. mile; cycling a 6-min. mile; ice or roller skating; gymnastics	6	60	180
walking a 12-min. mile; cycling a 5.5-min. mile; tennis-raquetball (singles)	7	70	210
walking an 11-min. mile; cycling a 5-min. mile; running in place; swimming (breast stroke laps—nonstop)	8	80	240
jogging a 10-min. mile; cycling a 4.3-min. mile; basketball; downhill skiing	11	110	330
running an 8.5-min. mile; boxing or wrestling; swimming (crawl stroke—nonstop)	13	130	390

From this it can be seen why exercise is an important part of obesity control. The greater the exercise, the greater the number of calories used and, if everything else remains unchanged, the greater the weight loss.

When considering caloric utilization, calorie intake must also be included. Just as caloric utilization has been studied, the caloric content of various foods and beverages has been well defined. Numerous books from the simple to the comprehensive are available. You may wish to refer to one of them. A representative list of selected foods and beverages along with calorie content follows. In order to illustrate for you the difference between high- and low-calorie foods, the list has been divided accordingly.

High		**Low**	
FOOD	CALORIES	FOOD	CALORIES
milk—whole (8 oz)	160	milk—skim (8 oz)	87
cheese—cheddar (1 oz)	115	chicken—broiled (3 oz)	115
cream (1 oz)	110	fish—broiled (3 oz)	140
cream—sour (2 oz)	160	peas (4 oz)	65
whipped (2 oz)	110	beans—lima (4 oz)	80
ice cream (one scoop)	300	green (4 oz)	45
eggs (two fried)	200	navy (4 oz)	80
bacon (three slices)	150	broccoli (4 oz)	46
steak (3 oz)	330	cabbage—raw (4 oz)	10
lamb chop (one)	400	carrots—raw (one)	10
pork chop (one)	370	celery (one stalk)	7
hamburger (one)	470	potato—baked (one)	80
cheeseburger (one)	560	tomato (one)	40
hot dog (one)	285	corn (one ear)	80
beef potpie (4¼″)	560	apple (one)	80
chili—canned (8 oz)	335	peach (one)	35
tuna fish sandwich (one)	290	orange (one)	65
peanut butter/jelly sandwich	390	grapefruit (one half)	45
candy—fudge (2 oz)	230	orange juice (8 oz)	88
chocolate (2 oz)	290	grapefruit juice (8 oz)	90
pie—apple (one slice)	350	bran flakes (4 oz)	55
cake—devil's food (one)	235	shredded wheat (4 oz)	60
cola (12 oz)	150	bread (one slice)	70
butter and margarine (1 tbs)	125	popcorn—no salt (one cup)	25
mayonnaise (1 tbs)	125		

It is imperative that you become knowledgeable about the caloric content of foods. It is only by so doing that you can become aware of the tremendous difference between numbers of calories in various foods.

The caloric rule of weight gain is simple. If you consume more calories than you utilize, it is stored as fat tissue. By the same token, if you use more calories than you take in, fat tissue will be used for energy and you lose weight. The magic number is 3,500. If you consume 3,500 more calories than you use, you will gain one pound. Conversely, if you use 3,500 more than ingested, you will lose one pound of fat tissue. This rule never changes. You can predict very accurately how much weight you are going to lose or gain based upon caloric intake and expenditure.

Creeping Obesity

One of the greatest problems with obesity is that it has a tendency to creep up on you. If you are a woman, can you recall how much you weighed when you were eighteen years old? For you men, can you remember your weight when you were twenty-five years old? Some authorities are of the opinion that your ideal body weight, regardless of your present age, should, for women, be the same as when you were eighteen years old and for men, the same as when twenty-five years old.

Unfortunately for most, body weight has a way of moving up with the passage of time. One reason for this is because as we get older our caloric requirements decline. From age twenty-five to forty, the amount of calories needed by the body declines 10 to 20 percent. As we advance from age forty to sixty-five, the amount of calories needed drops 20 percent. This means that if your caloric expenditure remains constant and you continue to eat exactly the same amount and kinds of food, you will *gain 3 pounds per year.* Over a ten-year period, *this is a total weight gain of 30 pounds and you have not increased your eating in any way.* Can you imagine what happens with the combination of reduction in exercise and an increase in eating habits?

It is imperative that you know and understand caloric content and utilization. Without this understanding, there can be no effective program for permanent weight loss. I want to give you several illustrations of how important it is to count calories.

There are 39 calories in a small pat of butter which you are served in a restaurant. If you are accustomed to eating butter and you eliminate just one pat of butter per meal, at the end of the month you will have eliminated 3,600 calories from your diet. One small, almost infinitesimal butter pat per meal means you will *lose 12 pounds in weight per year.* Now for the bad news. If you add one butter pat per meal, you will gain 12 pounds per year.

Let's say you drink milk—one glass of milk per meal. One glass of whole milk contains 180 calories. If you switch from whole to skim milk, you will reduce your calorie consumption by 7,200 calories per month. By this simple switch, you will *lose 24 pounds per year.*

I hope these several simple examples prove to you the importance of knowing and understanding the caloric content of foods and realizing that a minor change or elimination of a given food can add or take off many pounds.

You may say that a weight gain of a few pounds per year is not significant. If you gain a half pound per month, at the end of the year you have gained 6 pounds. Doesn't sound like much and it isn't, but the problem is that if you continue to gain this insignificant amount each year for five or ten or twenty years, you have gained, 30, 60, and 120 pounds, respectively.

Now perhaps you can reflect back to when you were eighteen or twenty-five years old and understand how easy it is for creeping obesity to sneak up on you. Before you know it, you have gained weight which you thought could be lost as easily as gained. The only problem with this kind of thinking is that taking it off once it accumulates is extremely difficult.

HOW AND WHY OBESITY IS HARMFUL

Of all the negative lifestyles that detract from high-level wellness, obesity is one of the most serious. Some feel it is *the* most serious. There are many authorities who are of the opinion that obesity is the most prevalent cause of premature death. It has been pointed out that "cutting down on the amount of food consumed is another way to cut down on premature death. If all the obesity in the population was eliminated, it would probably have the greatest impact on increasing life-span." This is what high-level wellness is all about—eliminating a negative lifestyle which will, in turn, reduce premature death and increase life-span. By assuming control over your problem of obesity and achieving and maintaining ideal body weight, you will achieve high-level wellness, feel better, and live longer.

How many times have you thought about going on a diet? How many times have you actually started on a diet? How many books have you read on diet programs? How many pounds have you lost and gained back? How many times have you wished you could lose weight and not gain it back?

Today you stand at a critical point in your life. I know that losing weight is important to you, perhaps one of the most important things in your life. Today you are starting on a program for weight reduction that cannot fail. Your goal and ideal body weight is now under your control and achievable. You probably wonder how I can be so sure. It's simple. Starting today, you are going to educate your mind to take command of your obesity problem.

Until now you have tried to regain control of your eating habits by ignoring mind function. This is why you have failed. In order to be a success with permanent weight loss, you must instruct and inform the mind as to exactly how and why obesity destroys vital organs and body systems. At the present time, your mind has no comprehension as to the harmful effects of being obese. Remember, the body cannot think. It will continue

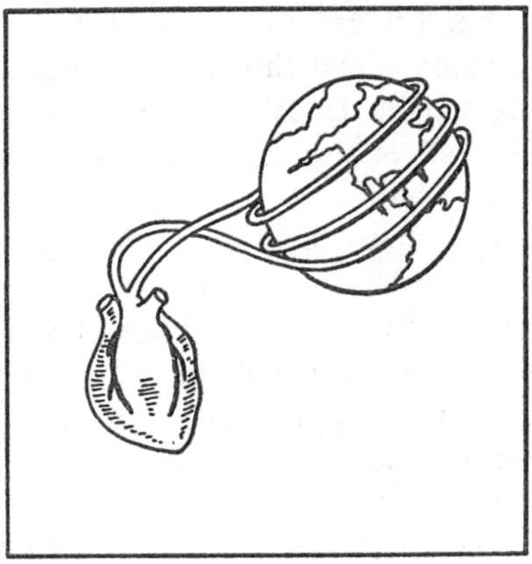

Normal circulation network (*66,000 miles*): Heart designed to pump blood through the circulatory system of an individual of ideal body weight.

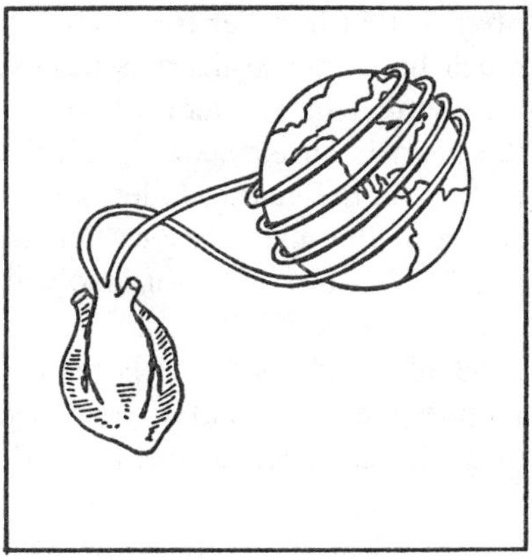

Obese circulation network (*88,000 miles*): In the obese individual the heart must pump blood thousands of extra miles.

to send out hunger signals with no consideration as to the devastating effects of overeating until the educated mind intervenes.

Following is the basic information you need to educate your brain and become involved in your program. Study it carefully and repeatedly until you know and comprehend exactly *how* and *why* obesity is harmful to vital organs and body systems. Learn *how* and *why* obesity causes premature death and prevents high-level wellness.

Obesity and Cardiovascular Disease

Being obese places a tremendous extra work load on the heart. It is estimated that the average person of normal weight has 66,000 miles of circulatory vessels in the body. In other words, if every artery, arteriole, capillary, venule, and vein were connected together in one continuous "tube," it would be 66,000 miles long—sufficient to stretch around the world three times! The heart is constantly pushing blood through this enormous circulatory system.

Fat tissue is no different from other body tissue in that every cell must receive oxygen and a variety of nutrients. Carbon dioxide and other waste products must be removed. The delivery and removal work is done by the blood through the circulatory system. There are hundreds of thousands of cells in each pound of fat tissue. Each cell must be serviced by the blood. Each extra pound of fatty tissue requires many additional miles of circulatory vessels. In the obese person, the heart is required to pump blood through hundreds, perhaps thousands, of miles of extra vessels. It is obvious that in order for the heart to accomplish extra work, it must work much harder. The heart is designed to pump blood through the circulatory system of a person of normal body weight. Under these conditions, the heart is an efficient machine. Obesity places a constant, never-relenting tax on the heart. Under the extra work load the heart deteriorates and is one of the main reasons that obesity is perhaps the most critical negative lifestyle or risk factor involved with cardiovascular diseases.

It is imperative that you be able to mentally visualize hundreds of extra miles of circulatory vessels required by your extra pounds of fatty tissue. Picture the extra labor your heart must perform to push your blood through this unbelieveable network of extra blood vessels.

The diagram to the left (on page 155) illustrates the approximately 66,000 miles of circulatory vessels in the body of a person of ideal weight. The heart can cope with this pumping job very efficiently. If you are male and approximately 6 feet tall, you should weigh about 155 to 160 pounds. If you weigh 200 pounds you are almost 25 percent overweight, which means your expanded circulatory vessels are equal to another circuit around the world. Your heart must push the blood an extra 22,000 miles. This is pictured to the right.

You wouldn't expect a Volkswagen engine to successfully power a Rolls-Royce automobile. Yet, if you are obese, this is the kind of performance you expect from your overworked heart.

Obesity and Hypertension

Hypertension (high blood pressure) is one of the most serious of the cardiovascular diseases. It is estimated by the American Heart Association that approximately 34 million people have hypertension. Half of this estimated number have the disease and don't know it. Hypertension is called the silent killer because in many instances there are no symptoms associated with it. It is estimated that one out of every three males have or will develop hypertension. This disease is one of the most important causes of a stroke or heart attack.

If you are prone to develop hypertension, it will be aggravated by obesity. Notice I did not say that obesity will cause hypertension, but if you have a tendency to develop the disease, your obesity will cause it to become clinically evident sooner and cause it to be more severe.

How and why does obesity cause hypertension to become worse? The main reason is basically physical. The fatty tissue surrounds the arteries and veins. The more obese you get, the more external pressure is applied to the blood vessels. This causes the diameter of the vessels to become smaller. The heart continues to pump with the same force, but since the diameter of the vessels is smaller, the pressure goes up.

The following illustrations picture for you the reaction of the arteries, capillaries, and veins of a person of normal body weight and the reaction of the circulatory system that is surrounded and compressed by fatty tissue. Since the blood in both illustrations is being pumped with equal force, it is easy to visualize *how* and *why* the pressure goes up because of the severe reduction in internal size of the circulatory vessels.

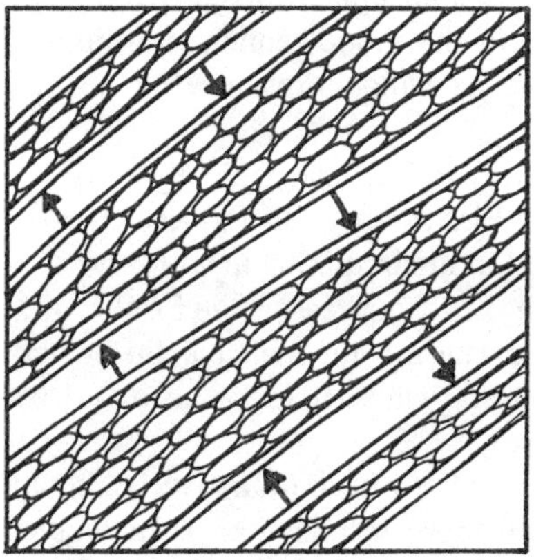

Ideal body weight: There is little or no fatty tissue to place unnatural pressure on the arteries.

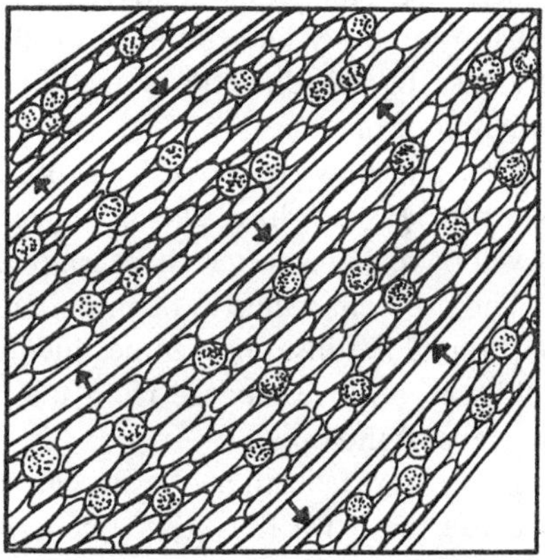

Obesity and hypertension: Fatty tissue compresses the arteries, causing blood pressure to increase.

You must develop the ability to picture and even feel your fatty tissue applying pressure on and compressing your arteries, capillaries, and veins. Develop a mental picture of your blood being compressed and moving under much greater pressure.

When a physician first diagnoses hypertension, if the patient is overweight, one of the standard recommendations is to lose weight. Often with significant weight loss, the hypertension either improves or disappears. The pressure being applied by the fatty tissue is gone and pressure returns to normal.

Obesity and Diabetes

In people who are 50 percent or more overweight, the incidence of diabetes is twelve times greater than for a person of normal body weight. Eighty percent of all diabetics are obese.

Just as with hypertension, it would probably not be correct to suggest that obesity causes diabetes, but if you are prone to develop the disease, being obese definitely causes it to become clinically active.

What is diabetes? A simple definition is "the body's inability to metabolize carbohydrates, which causes an elevation of glucose in the blood and urine." This elevation of glucose (a form of sugar) in the blood can lead to a variety of metabolic problems.

Insulin is normally secreted by the pancreas in response to the increase in blood glucose following the eating of a meal (another of the body's checks and balances systems). Insulin causes an uptake of glucose by the cells in the body and the level of glucose in the blood remains normal. In the case of the diabetic, something happens which prevents the normal function of insulin.

Why and how does obesity cause diabetes to become clinically evident? Several reasons have been suggested. First, when the obese person develops diabetes, often there is no reduction in circulating insulin.

The problem seems to be in the fact that for some reason the insulin or a portion of the insulin becomes ineffective. The incompetent insulin has no ability to remove glucose from the blood and cause it to be absorbed by the cells of the body.

Another reason that obesity causes diabetes to become active is simply because the extra fatty tissue cells require more insulin than is available. When this occurs, the organ that produces insulin becomes overworked, tired, and ineffective. Thus, glucose accumulates in the blood.

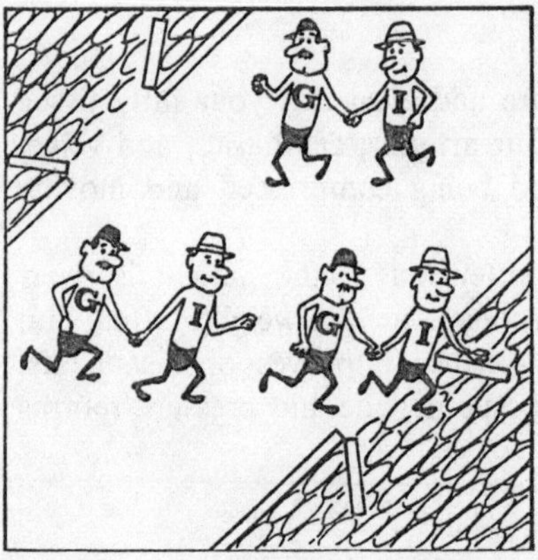

Normal weight: In an individual whose weight is ideal, there is sufficient effective insulin to keep the blood free of sugar (glucose).

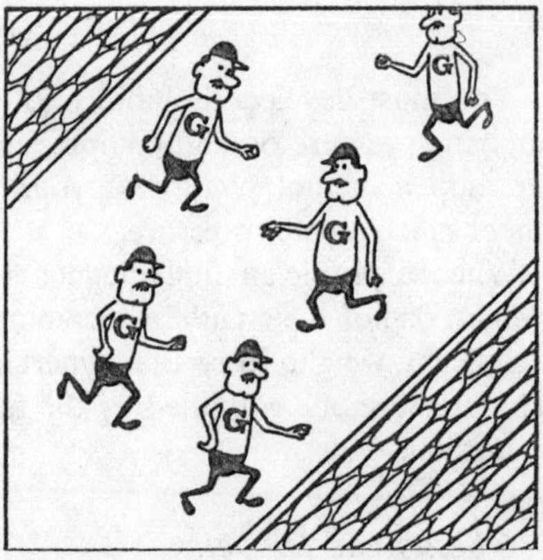

Obesity and diabetes: The obese individual requires more effective insulin than the body can produce and therefore sugar (glucose) accumulates in the blood.

On the left is an artist's concept of the utilization of glucose in a person of normal weight. There is a sufficient amount of effective insulin to cause cellular uptake of excess glucose causing the blood to be sugar-free. On the right is an illustration of an obese person in which the amount of insulin is insufficient and part of that which is available is ineffective. This results in an accumulation of glucose in the blood.

This entire explanation of how obesity is one of the prime complicating factors in diabetes may sound complex. If so, it's because it is complex. The main point for you to understand is that obesity can and will cause latent diabetes to become active. You must develop the ability to mentally visualize the extra insulin required by your excess fatty tissue. Get a picture of ineffective insulin not permitting the glucose in your blood to be absorbed by the cells. Develop an image of excess sugar in your blood and all the problems this can cause, such as blindness, poor circulation, cardiovascular problems, neurological problems, dermatological problems, and many more. What you need to do is saturate your mind with information about the relationship between obesity and diabetes and the disastrous effects it can have, destroying vital organs and body systems.

Obesity and Musculoskeletal Problems

The human skeleton is a fairly delicate structure. It and the muscular system form an efficient and durable combination which will last for many decades. The musculoskeletal system is designed to carry a certain amount of weight. While some extra weight may be tolerated, when a person becomes obese, the extra load placed on the musculoskeletal system is significant. In the case of pronounced obesity, it is very serious.

Obese people will have more problems with joint diseases, particularly of the knees and ankles. The reason for this is obvious. If an extra twenty, forty, or sixty pounds are being carried around and supported by the joints, they tend to wear out faster. These problems are especially true of the individual who is prone to arthritis. Since much of the extra weight is often carried around the middle of the body, it is not unusual for diseases of the hip joints to be seen more frequently in the obese person.

Individuals who are obese often will have more muscular problems, particularly in the lower back. When excessive weight is carried in the form of a "potbelly" or "bay window," it places an extremely heavy load on the large muscles of the lower back. Under such conditions, these muscles are very prone to strain and sprain.

It is difficult to provide you with a picture to illustrate the harmful effect your obesity has on your joints and muscles. Your obesity is obvious. You must learn to develop the mental picture of the extra weight, strain, and work load your extra weight places on your joints and muscles.

By constantly placing an extra work load on your joints and muscles, your obesity detracts from high-level wellness. The reason for this is simple. If you are constantly experiencing low-grade joint and muscle pain, you can never experience high-quality life and, hence, can never enjoy high-level wellness.

Miscellaneous Problems Associated with Obesity

Several other problems are associated with obesity which many never think about but are important.

Obese people have a much more difficult time in adjusting to a warm or hot environment. The body fat acts as insulation and holds body heat in. For this reason, the obese person will be much more uncomfortable in warm conditions than a person of normal body weight. This is why obese people perspire much more profusely. Some have suggested that in addition to being uncomfortable, this self-contained body heat may be a complicating factor in certain diseases.

Many surgeons think that obese patients, especially those who are severely obese, are a higher risk during major surgery. The reasons for this are that the heart may already be overworked, pulmonary problems may develop, and the physical aspect of performing the surgery may be more complicated and prolonged.

Obese persons usually have more problems in mobility. If you are carrying extra weight, it is more difficult to move around, climb up stairs, or get up out of a chair. These problems in mobility can prevent some from participating in certain activities which those of normal weight enjoy.

In summary, it can be said that obesity definitely detracts from high-level wellness, maximum longevity, and high-quality life.

You now have sufficient information on how and why obesity destroys your vital organs and body systems. Go back and reread the material in this chapter. You may wish to go to your library and study other materials on obesity and its effect on the body. But this book provides a basis for now. I want you to become your own expert on exactly how and why obesity is harmful to you and how and why it will cause premature death. Saturate your mind with this information. Convert the information into personal knowledge. Your mind is starving for a five-course meal of information. Feed your mind instead of your body.

Remember, your body-need–appetite regulator is adjusted to "eat all the time." The reason for this is that the mind is devoid of information and, therefore, overeating is an okay activity.

The solution to your obesity problem is simple. Feed the mind the proper information and new signals will start to be sent to the body. These new signals say: Obesity is harmful and here are the reasons why . . . ; obesity destroys vital organs and body systems and here are the reasons why . . . ; obesity inhibits high-quality life and here are the reasons why . . . ; obesity causes premature death and here are the reasons why . . .

When these signals are sent from mind to body, strange things start to happen. You will find that you will experience a "full" feeling after eating less food. You will find that the midmorning and midafternoon hunger pangs which previously drove you almost crazy will disappear. You will find that your desire for those foods that you have learned are high in calories will be lost. You will find that your urge for a midnight snack will be satisfied with a piece of fresh fruit. You will find that mild hunger pangs are something you really can tolerate and, in fact, enjoy as a feeling of accomplishment.

All of these things and others will occur without any conscious effort on your part. As you read this, you may be skeptical. You may say, "I have tried every diet that came along and have always failed." The reason you have failed is because you have never had a program that allowed you to regain control of your body-need–appetite regulator. Until now, your appetite has been like a moving ship without a rudder—no direction, no control—simply eat all the time.

After you totally indoctrinate the mind about the harmful effects of obesity, the signals are sent out to eat only when energy and nutrients are needed. Now your long-sought-after goal is at hand. You will start to lose weight. You will continue to lose weight until you have achieved a predetermined goal and you will maintain your ideal body weight for the rest of your extended and high-quality life. High-level wellness is at this moment in sight for you.

YOUR PERSONAL WEIGHT LOSS PLAN

You are now ready to review the program that will allow you to return to and maintain normal body weight. From now on, your mind will transmit the proper signals to return your appetite to normal. Remember, your problem is not in your stomach, but in your mind.

At the end of this chapter, you will find a list of ideas and tips that are useful adjuncts to your visualization program. In addition, several typical and representative menus are provided which give you a general idea of what a 1,500-calorie diet is like.

Step One: *Make your personal commitment to lose weight and never gain it back again.* Your commitment to *permanently* losing and maintaining ideal body weight is one of the most important you will ever make. You probably have made commitments to lose weight before. Perhaps you actually achieved your goal but soon regained all the lost weight. It doesn't matter how many times you have taken this roller-coaster ride. You are about to remove your excess weight for the last time.

The starting point of this process is your written commitment to a slimmer and trimmer body. You have already made the decision that obesity is the negative lifestyle you most want to eliminate.

I want you to carefully think through your personal commitment and determine *why* losing weight is so important. You must also know *how* important it is. How important is achieving permanent, ideal weight when compared to other activities in your life? Now you must write a summary of your thoughts. Your written commitment may be several sentences or pages in length. The number of words doesn't matter. The act of mental analysis and the written word is the important part. The main point is for you to *know* why this project is important and to issue written instructions so your mind will comprehend the importance.

Devote 100 percent of your efforts, energy, and concentration toward gaining control of your eating habits. By applying this total commitment and concentration, and total immersion effort, you will be amazed how quickly your desire for food and eating habits change. Sooner than you ever dreamed possible, you will have complete control over your problem of obesity and you will be proceeding with your program for the elimination of another negative lifestyle.

Step Two: *Study and review again all the material and data in this chapter that explains how and why obesity destroys your vital organs and body systems.* This step is the backbone of your program. I want you to become an expert in exactly how and why being obese causes premature death and how it prohibits high-quality life.

You must become aware of the widespread problem of obesity—how and why it may be the most significant factor causing premature death. Become convinced that you will die two years sooner for every ten pounds you are above normal weight. Learn about the almost inconceivable amount of extra circulatory vessels required by your excess fat. Comprehend the tremendous extra work load your heart must assume to pump blood through this additional mileage of circulatory vessels. Think about your heart as it must contract much harder with each beat.

Learn how and why obesity can precipitate hypertension (high blood pressure). Know how the fatty tissue exerts pressure on your veins and arteries, causing them to lose their elasticity and decreasing internal diameter. Understand why your blood moves through arteries and veins under higher pressure because of this. Become knowledgeable about the relationship between hypertension and having a stroke or heart attack.

Become familiar with all the data relative to the fact that diabetes is seen much more frequently in obese people. Learn exactly how and why this occurs. Learn how obesity is involved in causing diabetes to become symptomatic. Know about all the problems that are associated with excessive glucose in the blood.

Comprehend the unbelievable strain and stress that excessive weight places on joints and the muscle system. Think particularly of the ankle, knee, and hip joints. The extra weight you carry around your middle is supported to a large degree by the muscles of the lower back. Learn about this extra weight pulling and straining these muscles and how easy it is for fatigue and injury to occur.

Step Three: *Develop the ability to mentally visualize the disastrous effects obesity has on your vital organs and body systems.* The secret to your program for the elimination of obesity as a negative lifestyle is to convert all the new information and data you have into mental pictures. To this end, conceptual illustrations are provided in this chapter. They give a visual interpretation of the harmful effects of obesity on your vital organs and body systems.

You will notice that pairs of illustrations are used. One shows the effects of obesity, the other the same system in the individual of normal body weight.

You must study the illustrations until you can recall in minute detail what the harmful effects of obesity look like. Remember, this is what's going on inside your body. Next, be able to convert your mental pictures of your obesity-ravished system to the healthy, normally functioning system that you will enjoy after you have achieved your ideal body weight. It's this ability to create a picture of the devastating effects of obesity that causes new and different signals to be transmitted to your body. These new and different signals change your body regulators from constant hunger and desire for food to eating only where there is a body need for energy and nourishment. Constant, uncontrolled eating is no longer an okay activity and, therefore, is rejected.

You must be able to instantly visualize the miles of extra circulatory vessels required by your excessive fatty tissue—the extra work load placed on your heart—develop mental pictures of how and why your obesity can and will precipitate hypertension and diabetes. On your mental television, tune in pictures of the tremendous strain placed on joints and the muscle system. In summary, be able to develop vivid mental recall of exactly the effects of obesity on your body. Then be able to convert this mental kaleidoscope into pictures of your body systems after your weight has returned to normal.

Step Four: *Write a summary of everything you learn about how and why obesity is harmful to your vital organs and body systems.* When trying to learn new information or material, the most efficient method is to use as many of the senses as possible. For this reason, it is imperative that while learning how and why obesity is harmful, you write down everything you know.

As you write your summary, calculate the number of calories you require each day. Then estimate the number you consume daily. Figure out how many calories you should have in order to lose one to two pounds each week. Write a summary of the effect of obesity on the cardiovascular system. Write out in detail the relationship between obesity and hypertension and diabetes. Describe how and why obesity is involved in musculoskeletal problems.

You should feel free to improvise your own visualization illustrations. Using those in this chapter as a guide, draw your own interpretation of obesity causing damage to your vital organs and body systems. Then produce your drawings of how things will look after you have achieved ideal weight and obesity is no longer a problem.

Step Five: *Practice visualization programs every morning upon awaking, noon, evening, just before going to sleep, and every time there is an urge to eat.* Learning *how* to visualize and *when* to visualize are two completely different activities. One mistake that many make is not to organize a program or schedule for visualization. They think that the task is complete when the art of visualization is learned. They think that once learned, visualization comes automatically. Not so. You must have a definite, predetermined schedule so that visualization can and will take place every day at strategic times.

You should begin by associating your visualization schedule with established routine. You should train yourself that the first thought to enter your mind upon waking in the morning is your visualization program. Think through and visually study the harmful effects of obesity on your body. Do this before your mind becomes cluttered with other thoughts of the day's activities and problems. You will find that, at first, other thoughts will enter your mind. However, after several days of conscientiously placing top priority on your visualization program, it will become automatic. It will become the subject of your first thoughts of the day with no effort on your part. So, lie there reviewing your mental television of the harmful effects of obesity. This will set your day. Your mind will be oriented upon arising to adjust your appetite to moderate eating for the entire day.

As you become involved with your visualization program, try and tie in with other daily routines. If you take a morning mini-meal break, always practice your visualization program thirty minutes before break time. Do the same for the afternoon break. It will amaze you how you will be completely satisfied with a glass of grapefruit juice instead of coffee and several doughnuts.

If you work outside the home or if you work at home, train yourself to visualize thirty minutes before the evening meal. Since for most people this is the largest meal of the day, it is imperative that you visualize in order to obtain control of your appetite. Remember, once the brain understands how and why obesity causes premature death, signals to reduce and control the appetite are sent out. The entire process is out of your control. The end result is that, for the first time, perhaps in years, your appetite responds to body needs instead of habit.

Probably the best and most effective time for visualization is immediately before going to sleep. The mind is very active during sleep. It can learn when you are asleep or when you are awake. If you prime your thought process with your visualization program just before going to sleep, it will be reinforced and you can be assured it will be the first item to occur to you upon awaking.

Above all, you must condition yourself to automatically visualize *every time* you have the urge to eat. It will surprise you how visualization will stop your hunger pangs in their tracks. Your mind at last has something to think about instead of eating.

Once you learn how to visualize, you will do so unconsciously. Different phases of your program will flash across your mind at unscheduled times. This is great! When you reach this point of unanticipated or unplanned visualization, the program is a part of you. You have it made. Your body is saying, "Take control. Tell me why I shouldn't eat so much."

Step Six: *Determine and write down a schedule or target date whereby you will accomplish your predetermined weight reduction.* You must have a schedule for weight loss. Your actual weight loss will be determined by a combination of reduction in calories and increase in exercise, so every individual case will respond differently. However, I want to caution you against a weight reduction program that is too fast. You did not become obese in a month, and you cannot expect to correct your problem in a month.

What you are searching for is a permanent change in eating habits. Even with your program for visualization, it will take a period of time to readjust eating habits that have been out of adjustment for years. One of my basic concerns about diets that promise you will lose 20 pounds in two weeks is that they do nothing to alter basic eating habits. No program can alter eating habits that fast. I have no doubt that some can lose the 20 pounds, but since eating habits have not been changed, they will quickly be gained back.

A reasonable and achievable goal is to lose 2 pounds per week. You may say: "With all this conversation about how effective this program is, why go so slow—only two pounds per week?" First, I am most interested in a safe program for weight reduction. Second, I want this to be your last effort at a weight reduction program. For these reasons, a 2-pound-per-week reduction is ideal. If you think this is too slow, I would remind you that in three months—just ninety days—you will have lost 26 pounds. In six months you will have lost 52 pounds. So, it can be seen that this program is not as slow as it may seem, yet it is a program that allows you to change your eating habits over a period of time. This allows for permanent weight loss.

The main point is for you to have a specific weekly goal for weight reduction: 2 pounds a week or less. The mind will respond best when a definite goal is involved. Your educated and visualization-oriented mind will always respond to your desires. Educate your mind, visualize, and move out of the way.

It is absolutely imperative that you write your goals down. Just as when accumulating your basic information as to how and why negative lifestyles are harmful, you must have a written record of your goal. You must challenge your mind in writing, give it something to shoot for. The challenge is a command to the mind. A command in writing always demands more reaction than a verbal or mental order.

After you issue your written objective, your goal is totally within your control. To lose 10 pounds, 40 pounds, 55 or 100 pounds—it makes no difference. According to your written goal, your desires will be accomplished.

Step Seven: *Develop a vivid mental picture of you at your predetermined weight.* You have now reached the point where you know how to develop your program for visualization. You have determined your weight-loss goal. Only one factor remains. You must provide the mind with an image of what you will look like after you have achieved your weight-loss goal. The mind responds to this type of positive suggestion. Thus, you must visualize yourself already having achieved your goal.

Remember, it is a fact that you become what you think about! You are the sum total of your thought processes. For this reason, the last element of your weight reduction program is a preconceived visual picture of you at your ideal weight. Every time you practice visualization, finish it off with you as you will soon look and be.

In anticipation of the accomplishment of your goal, go out now and purchase yourself a piece of wearing apparel that you will wear after you are at your ideal weight. Make it something simple—perhaps a new belt or a blouse. Regardless of how ridiculous it may seem now, it is only a matter of time until it will be a perfect fit.

Providing your brain with a visual goal to shoot for is an important element of the program. Don't neglect it.

That's it. You now have at your disposal your program for achieving your ideal body weight. If applied exactly as outlined, it never fails. Regardless of the number of weight-loss failures you have experienced, this is not one of them. The reason for this is that now, for the first time, you have brought your thought processes into play. You have, for the first time, a program that provides a readjustment of your body regulators so that overeating is no longer an okay activity and therefore is to be rejected. Normal body weight is possible and achievable.

If you are looking ahead, you may be wondering about maintaining your newfound body weight. Just as visualization can help you achieve ideal body weight, it can also help you maintain it forever. The main point for you to remember is that you *must not* stop your visualization exercises once you have obtained your goal. You should continue your program indefinitely. Every time you have an urge to increase your eating habits, any time there is an urge to eat when not hungry, any time there is a desire for high-calorie foods, VISUALIZE! It's your answer to obtaining a slender body and a life of contentment, happiness, and self-satisfaction. You now have available everything required to know HOW TO GET YOUR WEIGHT DOWN STARTING NOW!

ADDITIONAL HELPFUL HINTS

At the end of each chapter you are provided with a brief outline of practical information, tips, and hints that are intended to supplement your visualization program. When used in conjunction with visualization, they will help you eliminate your negative lifestyle.

A number of suggestions are provided that will enable you to manage your calories. You will also find a representative and typical 1,500-calorie diet. This will give you a general idea of what a diet of this type is like.

1) Because of the close association between losing weight and good nutrition, you may find it beneficial to read chapter 6 before starting on your program to achieve ideal weight.

2) Be calorie-conscious. Become an expert on those foods and beverages that are extremely low in calories. Do this for regular and snack foods. Build your diet around them.

3) Don't be overanxious and try to lose too much weight too fast. Maximum loss should not exceed 2 pounds per week. It took you years to become obese. It will take a little time to correct the problem.

4) Determine the number of calories you should consume each day in order to provide energy requirements. If you want to lose 2 pounds per week, you must reduce your intake by 1,000 calories per day.

5) Get in the habit of counting calories at the grocery store. *Don't buy* foods and beverages that are high in calories. If you don't have it in the kitchen, you can't eat it.

6) Before each meal, take five minutes and *relax*. Being tense and anxious makes you eat faster and more food.

7) Take small portions; do not accept seconds.

8) *Take smaller bites*. Cut your food in portions one half the size you are accustomed to. Learn to take half-size portions onto your fork and spoon.

9) *EAT SLOWLY*. This is one of the most important tips I can give you. Put your fork or spoon down after each bite. By so doing, the stomach expands more slowly and you will experience a longer-lasting feeling of being full. When you eat fast, the calories go down in an uncontrolled way.

10) Never eat while preoccupied. If you are watching television, reading, working, drinking, or talking, you lose track of the food and calories consumed. When eating, concentrate exclusively on eating.

11) Convince your subconscious mind that you should never eat while standing, walking, or riding in a car. Eat only at mealtime, when seated at a table.

12) Don't be concerned about wasting food. You may have been taught never to waste food. It's better to save or throw away excess food than to eat it. When you consume food and calories beyond your preestablished limits, you waste your health and body.

13) When you get the urge to eat between meals, go for a walk or become involved in some other form of exercise. This will direct your mind away from the hunger and at the same time burn calories.

14) When you reach for a between-meal snack, stop, wait for five minutes, then ask yourself if you are really hungry.

15) If you know in advance that you are going to a big meal, plan for it. Place a *special reduction* on calorie intake for several days prior to the event. Eat one or two pieces of dry dark toast or a raw carrot or piece of fresh fruit thirty minutes before the meal is served. You will be surprised how this brings your appetite under control.

16) Don't take appetite-suppressant drugs. They are a crutch and do nothing to change your basic eating habits. In addition, they can cause dangerous side effects.

17) Keep a calorie diary so you can write down the number of calories you consume each day.

18) Concentrate on getting a good quantity of fiber in your diet. High-fiber foods are more filling and keep hunger away longer. They are usually ultra-low in calories.

19) Take a photograph of yourself in a bathing suit, as you begin your diet. Take additional pictures at regular intervals as you make progress. After you have achieved your goal, use the original photograph to instruct your subconscious mind of what you never want to look like again.

20) Always have low-calorie snack foods available. This can include fresh-cut raw vegetables (carrots, cabbage, celery, radishes) and fresh fruit (apples, oranges, grapefruit, peaches, pineapple, bananas). Dry dark toast is excellent. Homemade bran muffins (use one fourth the suggested sugar) are good. Fruit juices can curb the appetite with minimal calories. Popcorn that is popped without oil and no salt is a highly nutritious snack with very few calories.

21) Do not allow junk foods in your home. This includes all kinds of chips, pretzels, nuts, cookies, doughnuts, cakes and pastries, pies and ice cream. You can destroy a full day of successful dieting with one junk food session.

22) Increase your exercise by doing the following:

- Use the stairs instead of the elevator or escalator.
- Start to walk more and ride less.
- When walking, do it briskly.
- Don't sit any more than is necessary.
- Get out of bed early in the morning.

In order to achieve your goal, you must decrease caloric intake and increase exercise. Since caloric reduction is mandatory, the following two daily menus will give you an idea of what a 1,500-calorie diet is like.

1,500-Calorie (approx.) Diet

Breakfast

½ cup orange juice
½ cup all-bran cereal
½ dark English muffin
1 cup skim milk
1 cup decaffeinated coffee or decaffeinated tea

Lunch

2¼ cups tossed salad
1 tbs salad dressing (low cal)
1 slice whole-grain bread
1 small apple
1 cup skim milk

Dinner

3 oz baked chicken (no skin)
½ cup brown rice
½ cup green beans
10 fresh strawberries
1 cup decaffeinated coffee or decaffeinated tea

Breakfast

½ grapefruit
½ cup oatmeal (not instant)
1 slice whole-grain bread
1 cup skim milk
1 cup decaffeinated coffee or decaffeinated tea

Lunch

2 oz low-fat cottage cheese
2 slices fresh or unsweetened pineapple
1 slice whole-grain bread
1 cup skim milk

Dinner

3 oz fish (baked or broiled)
1 small baked potato (plain, or 1 tbs low-fat yogurt)
½ cup broccoli
1 small orange
1 cup decaffeinated coffee or decaffeinated tea

8. HOW TO MODERATE YOUR DRINKING—OR QUIT COMPLETELY IF YOU WISH

"O God, that men should put an enemy in
their mouths to steal away their brains!
That we should, with joy, pleasance, revel
and applause, transform ourselves into beasts!"
OTHELLO, Act II, Scene 3

The annual per capita consumption of alcohol in the United States is 2.7 gallons of absolute ethyl alcohol for each person fourteen years and older. This amounts to 691 cocktails or beers or glasses of wine per person per year. There are approximately 10 million adult problem-drinkers and an additional 3.3 million between the ages of fourteen and seventeen. Alcoholism in all its ramifications is the third leading cause of death in the United States. In one of our largest cities, liver cirrhosis is the third leading cause of death in the 25- to 65-year-old group. One third of all traffic injuries and one half of all traffic fatalities are alcohol-related. Alcohol is involved in the majority of crimes of rape, assault, and homicide. One third of all suicides are alcohol-related. Excessive drinking has been implicated in child abuse, child molesting, and marital violence. Dr. William C. Menninger has said, "If alcoholism were a communicable disease, a national emergency would be declared."

Hundreds, perhaps thousands, of books have been written on the problems of alcoholism. *This is not one of them.* Alcoholism is an illness, a serious illness. One usually requiring a multidisciplined medical approach in order to achieve improvement and constant reinforcement and encouragement for a lasting cure. For the alcoholic or alcohol-dependent person, therapy, counseling, and treatment beyond that found in this book are

Snacks

Morning: 1 small orange

Afternoon: carrot sticks

Night: 2 cups popcorn (no butter or salt)

Snacks

Morning: 1 small banana

Afternoon: 2 small celery stalks

Night: 1 slice dark dry toast and ½ cup skim milk

If you are male and should have approximately 2,700 calories per day and consume a diet similar to this, you will have a daily deficit of slightly over 1,000 calories and should lose about 2 pounds per week. For the female who should have about 2,000 calories daily for body energy, this diet will provide a caloric deficit of approximately 500 calories each day. You will lose about one pound each week. If you wish to lose at a faster rate, you should decrease caloric intake to below 1,500 calories each day. All of this assumes your exercise pattern remains constant. If you increase caloric expenditure through exercise, you will make faster progress.

required. I am not suggesting the programs and concepts presented here will not be useful in assisting the alcoholic to achieve a cure, but I want to be sure that this program is not used to the exclusion of in-depth therapy.

This program for high-level wellness is designed for the social drinker, the escape drinker, the pleasure drinker, the drinker who asks, "Why am I drinking so much?", or "Are my drinking habits harmful to me?", or "Should I be drinking as much as I do?" This program is for the millions of people who drink, sometimes in large amounts and frequently, and really don't know why; for the millions who walk into a bar, jump up on a stool, start drinking and stare straight ahead without conversation or interaction with another person; for the millions of people who wake up the morning after with a throbbing head or sick stomach, go to the office feeling like warmed-over death, and say, "I'm never going to do that again"; this program is for the individual who says, "I want to cut back on my drinking" or "I really want to stop drinking."

Everyone who drinks has one thing in common, the ingestion of alcohol, so let's take a brief look at alcohol itself. The first point I want to convince you of is that *alcohol is a drug.* It is the most commonly used drug in the history of man and in the world today. Its widespread and universally accepted use has blurred the realization that this mind-altering substance is, in reality, a drug with devastating effects.

There are a number of organic chemical compounds called alcohols. Some of these are commonplace in our everyday lives. From a chemical point of view, the simplest of the alcohols is methyl alcohol or methanol. This is the alcohol that we call antifreeze and put in the radiator of the automobile to keep it from freezing. If you drank pure methanol, you would become irreversibly blind, as it has an affinity for attacking and destroying the optic nerve. Larger amounts of methanol are lethal. Another alcohol familiar to all is isopropyl alcohol, which we know as "rubbing" alcohol. Ingestion of rubbing alcohol causes violent sickness. The alcohol that is consumed on a regular basis is ethyl alcohol or ethanol. This is the alcohol found in beer, wine, and liquor. From a chemical point of view, the only difference between each of these three alcohols is a single methyl group.

Alcohol is a foreign compound and a toxic material to the human body. It is one of several items—water is another—that require no digestion when they are consumed. It passes directly into the blood through the stomach and small intestine. Because no digestion is required, alcohol is carried to the brain within several heartbeats after a swallow. It is the effect and influence that alcohol has on the brain which causes people to do strange things. What are some of these strange activities? Alcohol makes the meek become boisterous, the introvert to become extravert, the quiet to become verbose. It can cause one to momentarily forget worries and concerns. Sometimes alcohol will cause the peacemaker to want to fight. Occasionally it makes people fall down and sometimes they are not able to remember what happened the night before.

The reaction to alcohol varies greatly from one person to another. It would serve no purpose to try to explain why this occurs, because you know how you respond and that's the important thing. Your response to alcohol is based upon its depressant or anesthetizing (numbing) effect on certain portions of the brain. Many people think that alcohol is a stimulant, because of initial mood changes. This is easy to understand, because these mood changes (more talkativeness, less concern with problems, or becoming more outgoing) seem to be uplifting. What actually happens is that the portion of the brain responsible for inhibitions is anesthetized. Once this part of the brain is put to sleep, you appear to become more relaxed and carefree.

Let's consider what happens with the first drink. Alcohol is metabolized or burned and broken down in the body at a fairly constant rate. If you drink faster than it can be metabolized, the drug starts to accumulate in the blood and the concentration increases. Body size has something to do with this increase in concentration. The larger the person, the slower the increase in the concentration of alcohol in the blood. A 150-pound person can metabolize about three fourths of an ounce of alcohol per hour. This means if you drink:

1½ ounces of 100-proof whiskey, or

18 ounces of beer (1½ cans), or

one 5-ounce glass of wine

over a period of one hour, you will never have an accumulation of alcohol in the blood and, therefore, will not experience the feeling of inebriation that is the result of the brain's being anesthetized.

Most people I know will not stretch a single cocktail or beer or glass of wine over a period of an hour, so what happens as larger amounts of alcohol are consumed?

Following is a chart that shows the concentration of alcohol in the blood caused by a given number of drinks. To the right are mood changes that may be caused by these amounts of alcohol. It is important to realize that the mood changes are based on average reactions. Different variables are involved due to individual responses to the effect of the anesthetized brain. In the chart, a drink refers to one ounce of 100-proof whiskey, one beer, or one medium glass of wine.

Drinks/hr.	Blood level	Mood changes
1–2	0.04%	Flushing of skin, inhibitions start to go, heart speeds up, carefree
3–4	0.05%*	Judgment slower, dizziness, coordination starts to become affected
5–6	0.10%**	Reaction time slowed, speech a little fuzzy, vision a bit blurred
6–8	0.16%	Staggering, seeing double, loss of balance
15–20	0.40%	Unconsciousness, pupils dilated, clammy skin
20–25	0.50%	Alcoholic poisoning, death

* Legal definition of being under the influence for most states.
** Legal definition of intoxication for most states.

HOW MUCH ALCOHOL FOR YOU?

Before starting on your program to eliminate excessive alcohol from your lifestyle, let's consider: *What's excessive consumption?* This is a difficult question for several reasons. Individuals tolerate alcohol differently. For millions of people, any amount of alcohol is too much. Falling into this category are those who simply cannot stop after one or two drinks. One or two lowers their inhibitions, makes them feel so good that they are going to have another, then another, and so on. On the other hand, you have the drinker who can stop by the local bar, have two draft beers, and leave—no more drinking for the day.

Where do you fit into this spectrum of drinking? Have you ever thought about how much you drink? That's the starting point. Starting now, take a personal inventory of the amount of alcohol you drink. Do you consume alcohol every day? Do you have an alcoholic drink with lunch? Do you drink during the day on weekends? How much alcohol do you drink each day? How many quarts or half gallons or six-packs, or bottles of wine do you buy weekly? Get a handle on the amount of alcohol you consume because *you are the one who must decide if it's excessive.* I cannot tell you whether you should eliminate alcohol completely or reduce the amount.

One of your responsibilities in eliminating excessive alcohol as a negative lifestyle is to establish your goal, either total elimination or reduction.

While I cannot establish your goal, I can provide information that may be useful as a guideline. The following definitions are usually accepted:

Heavy Drinker

- Has at least one drink daily and three or more drinks five times per week.
- Has at least one drink per day and four or more drinks three times per week.
- Has seven or more drinks several times each month.

Moderate Drinker

- Drinks almost every day, having at least one, but usually two drinks.
- Has three or four drinks once or twice a week.
- Drinks several times per month and has three or four, but sometimes five or six drinks.

Light Drinker

- Has not more than one drink several times a week.
- Has no more than three drinks several days per month.

Be very honest with yourself and determine if you are a heavy, moderate, or light drinker. Most people have a tendency to downgrade themselves. That is, they don't want to admit they are heavy drinkers. If you are going to successfully change or modify drinking habits, you must know where you are when you start.

The safest amount of alcohol is no alcohol. It would be easy to make this recommendation and proceed immediately to the program on how to eliminate alcohol from your lifestyle. I try this, and immediately lose most people.

After conducting hundreds of Wellness Seminars both in the corporate setting as well as for the community, I have come to several conclusions.

First, you must remember, we are not dealing with alcoholics or alcohol-dependent persons. We are working with the person who might range anywhere from the heavy to the light social drinker. There seems to be a pattern. The heavy and moderate social drinker wants to reduce the amount of alcohol consumed and the light social drinker often wants to eliminate it entirely from his or her lifestyle. The heavy and moderate drinkers are adamant—they don't want to stop drinking completely, just reduce the amount consumed. Any conversation about total elimination of alcohol and they are not interested.

I have had heavy and moderate drinkers tell me they can go on the latest fad diet which prohibits alcohol for weeks, perhaps a month or two. During this time, they abstain, but when the desired weight is lost, they are going to resume drinking.

It is because of real-life situations like these that this program is designed to accomplish one of two goals—either complete elimination of alcohol or the elimination of excessive alcohol consumption. If you, at this time, are against the total elimination of alcohol from your lifestyle, I would rather see you sharply reduce your consumption for the rest of your life than make no change at all. Something interesting often happens when a person who is against total elimination of alcohol is successful in reducing alcohol consumption over a period of time. Once the weekly consumption falls below a certain point, this individual, *on his or her own,* will often eliminate alcohol completely. This two-step approach to the elimination of alcohol as a negative lifestyle is not planned as such, but it does occur.

I have searched the literature to determine if there is an accepted standard recommendation for the upper levels of safety for alcohol consumption. Dr. Morris Chafitz, the former Director of the National Institute on Alcohol Abuse and Alcoholism, has suggested that for the average healthy adult the absolute top level of safe drinking is a maximum of 1.5 ounces of pure alcohol per twenty-four hours. This is three cocktails, three beers, or three medium-sized glasses of wine. Remember, this is the absolute maximum. If you consume amounts in excess of this, you are probably causing serious damage to your vital organs and body systems.

Another very important factor that must be considered as you establish your new, reduced alcohol program is to understand the necessity for not drinking every day. The liver metabolizes alcohol. This is not an easy task, because alcohol is a foreign substance. The consequences of subjecting the liver to daily alcohol metabolism is discussed in detail later in this chapter. Don't drink every day! You should have a period of at least forty-eight consecutive hours each week when you consume no alcohol. Others have suggested you abstain for one week out of each month. The main point is, give the liver a period of rest and relaxation from the difficult task of alcohol metabolism.

HOW DRY I AM!

I am probably more qualified to write this chapter than any other in this book. At one time, due to my busy schedule, I was a heavy social drinker.

One thing that helped me eliminate excessive alcohol from my lifestyle was: I started running in the evening, after work and before dinner. By so doing, I rediscovered a basic law of physics. It is impossible to be in two places at the same time. Being on the roads, running from 5:30 to 6:30 P.M., prevents one from being at home or in the local bar having two or three martinis.

At the same time, I was learning everything possible about how and why excessive alcohol is harmful to vital organs and body systems. In essence, I applied the exact same program and principles which I am going to describe to you. Did it work? I think so. Have I completely eliminated alcohol? No. I never drink hard liquor but will have an occasional beer or a glass of wine.

There are several advantages to be derived from eliminating or reducing alcohol consumption which are often overlooked. Two of them have to do with weight control. Alcohol is the most powerful appetite stimulant known to man. The custom of alcohol before a meal goes back to the Roman Empire when the population was intent upon gorging themselves, with no consideration for nutrition or weight control. Their main objective was to eat as much as possible. Alcohol was consumed before the meal with the desire of increasing the appetite to maximum levels. Our present-day "drinks before dinner" routine represents one of the most astonishing paradoxes of our generation. Millions of people are devoted to the body beautiful, maintaining proper weight and reducing food consumption, and yet, they have several drinks thirty minutes before dinner. This accomplishes the exact opposite of what they are striving for, appetite stimulation instead of appetite control and weight reduction or maintenance.

In addition to appetite stimulation, alcohol itself is very high in calories. The average cocktail, beer, or glass of wine contains approximately 150 to 180 calories. That may not sound like much, but nine cocktails, beers, or glasses of wine mean an extra half pound of body fat. At the beginning of this chapter, it was pointed out that the per capita consumption of alcohol is 691 cocktails, beers, or glasses of wine per year. If you are average and consume this number of drinks, the alcohol itself will add 124,380 calories to your diet each year. If you do not in some way burn these extra alcohol calories, they are converted to 35 pounds of extra body weight.

PREMATURE DEATH

The problems of excessive consumption of alcohol have been noted for thousands of years. Alcohol, as we know it, was discovered in Eurasia in what we now know as China and Egypt about five thousand years ago. There are numerous references to wine in the earliest Western and Chinese literature. Although rare, wine was available during the Trojan

War (1300 B.C.). The legend of Bacchus came into being around this time.

By the time of Christ, wine was a customary drink, particularly at ceremonies. The consumption of wine had become so sophisticated that the Bible refers to "good" and "bad" wine. Few references to wine exist in the Old Testament except that Noah and Abraham's nephew Lot had a tendency to overimbibe.

Today, the alcohol industry is a multibillion-dollar business. It is virtually impossible to pick up a national magazine and not be bombarded with attractive advertisements expounding the virtues of a particular brand of whiskey, wine, or beer. No sporting event can be watched on television without being informed which beer is best or why a particular wine is to be preferred.

Consumption of excessive alcohol as a negative lifestyle is very different from all other negative lifestyles. Let me explain. The majority of people who smoke want to quit. Almost all who are obese want to lose weight. Nearly everyone would like to become involved in a program of regular exercise. Everyone would like to be able to better cope with stress. Most would like to consume the best possible diet. With alcohol, it seems to be different. Excessive alcohol is a widely accepted lifestyle.

The most basic fact you must realize about consumption of excessive alcohol is its role in premature death. It has been pointed out that, according to averages, *when a thirty-year-old heavy drinker is compared with a thirty-year-old light drinker, the heavy drinker will die eight years sooner*. Excessive alcohol can take eight years off your life. In addition, there is no other negative lifestyle which so totally destroys the possibility for high-quality life.

WHY DO YOU DRINK?

I have asked hundreds of people why they drink excessively. The majority don't really know. The basic reason is simply that you are missing the basic information as to how and why excessive alcohol destroys vital organs and body systems. At the present time, the signals that are transmitted from mind to body have your body regulators set so that excessive alcohol is an okay activity. The body can't think. It will continue to attempt to metabolize any quantity of alcohol. The mind does not have sufficient information to change the signals and inform the body that excessive alcohol is harmful.

If you fall into this group of not knowing why you drink, what you must do is become your own expert on exactly how and why excess alcohol is harmful. After you have thoroughly indoctrinated the mind, a new set of signals will be sent. This time, the messages indicate that alcohol is no longer acceptable or is acceptable only in limited quantities. Then you will experience an adjustment in your alcohol regulators. Alcohol in excessive amounts will no longer be acceptable.

If you don't truly want to reduce or eliminate alcohol consumption, don't become involved in this program, because once your mind understands the harmful effects of alcohol, it will not tolerate excess amounts. The mind *will not* be a party to any activity understood to be harmful to the body. Once you have the basic knowledge, then employ visualization, your alcohol consumption is beyond your conscious control.

WHY AND HOW EXCESS ALCOHOL IS HARMFUL

Following is the basic information you need to inform your mind how and why excessive alcohol is harmful to vital organs and body systems. Study the material and illustrations carefully. Become your own expert and you will be amazed how easy it is to eliminate or reduce your consumption of alcohol.

Alcohol and the Brain

Alcohol in any quantity (one drink) causes the red cells of the blood to become sticky and clump together. Following is an illustration showing the difference between alcohol-free blood and that which is alcohol-contaminated.

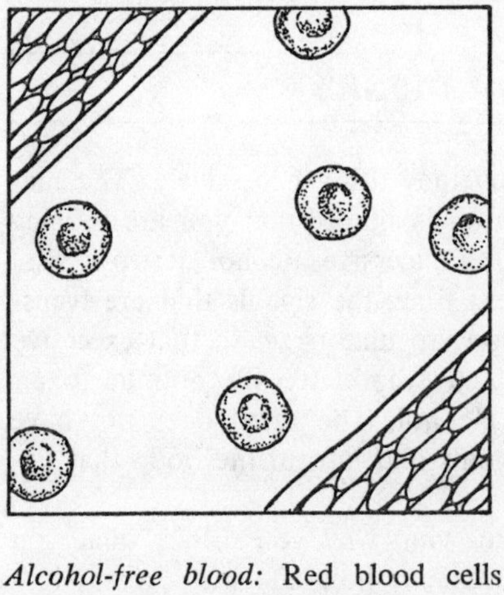

Alcohol-free blood: Red blood cells move freely, carrying oxygen to all parts of the body.

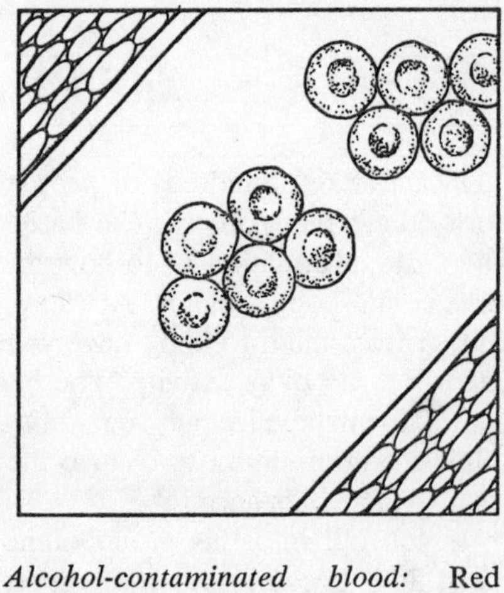

Alcohol-contaminated blood: Red blood cells clump together, slowing the blood flow.

On the left are the red blood cells moving freely through an artery. This blood is free of alcohol. On the right are red blood cells which are clumped together. This clumping is referred to as sludging and is caused by alcohol in the blood.

In the larger arteries, this is probably not a major problem. Oxygen release from the blood to the tissue takes place at the capillaries. Here is where the problem occurs. The capillaries are very small (and are referred to as the microcirculation). Often the clusters of sludged red cells are larger than the diameter of the small capillaries. This results in blockage and no blood flow. When this occurs, the cells in that area die from oxygen starvation. This happens throughout the body when the alcohol is consumed. Alcohol kills body cells by the hundreds of thousands. In most parts of the body, this is not a major event because cells can regenerate. Once the alcohol is out of the system, sludging stops and adequate oxygen flow returns. Not so with the brain. Brain cells do not regenerate. When they die from lack of oxygen at the capillary level due to red cell sludging, that minute portion of the brain is dead forever.

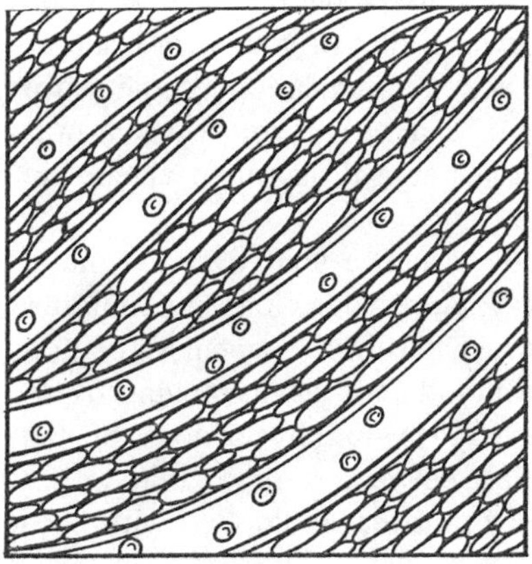

A brain capillary: Alcohol-free blood allows the free movement of red blood cells and the delivery of maximum amounts of oxygen to brain cells.

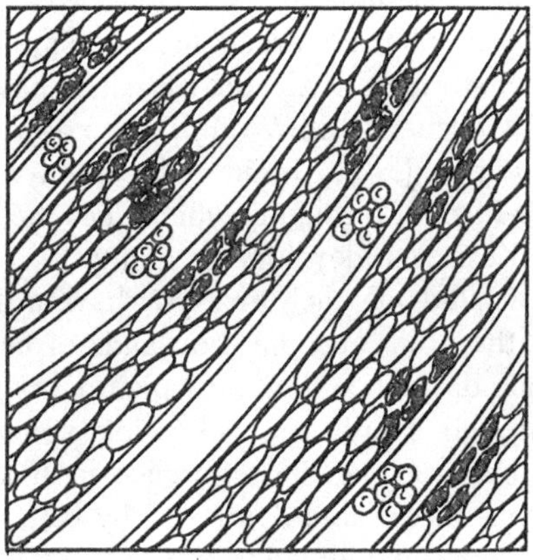

Alcohol influence: Red blood cell sludging causes blockage. Due to lack of oxygen, the brain cells die.

On the left is a capillary network at the brain level showing alcohol-free red blood cells flowing freely and releasing oxygen to surrounding brain cells. On the right can be seen red blood cell sludging, completely stopping blood flow. With inadequate blood flow and oxygen release, surrounding brain cells die and will not be regenerated.

Some say that alcohol-related red blood cell sludging brain damage is really not important because, after all, the brain is made up of billions of cells. What they fail to point out is that this brain cell damage is cumulative. If alcohol consumption is infrequent, they probably are correct—the total damage done is slight. But if it's chronic and in higher amounts, the results are pronounced. In this case, the damage to the brain is so advanced that it can be seen on gross examination (without a microscope) at autopsy. Often the pathologist will see brain lesions in the form of varicose veins, particularly in the area of the hypocampus. This probably explains why a lifetime of high alcohol consumption results in a memory deficiency.

There can be no high-level wellness along with excessive consumption of alcohol. When you drink beyond the boundaries of moderation, you are committing cerebral suicide. When you are knowingly and willingly killing thousands of brain cells daily over a twenty-, thirty-, perhaps fifty-year period, the end result is a complete annihilation of a high-quality intellectual life.

When you practice your visualization program to eliminate or reduce your consumption of alcohol, I want you to think of the destructive action of alcohol at the organ and body system level. Think of your own brain as a separate entity. You will then have a better appreciation of the harm that occurs to it. Would you knowingly take a pill if you knew it was going to destroy brain cells? Then why consume a drug called alcohol in the form of a cocktail which does the same thing?

You must develop the ability to mentally visualize your own red blood cells sludging each time you have a drink. Picture your clogged capillaries in the brain and the thousands of cells which die from oxygen starvation each day. Then you must picture your red blood cells clean, moving freely through capillaries, delivering abundant oxygen to all portions of the brain. Imagine the difference in the feeling between a brain that is oxygen-starved and dying cell by cell, and a brain that is flooded with oxygen and functioning to full capacity.

Alcohol and the Blood

Next to the brain, the liver is the most complex organ in the body. It is the liver that breaks down (metabolizes) everything that is ingested. The liver is very efficient when metabolizing carbohydrates, fats, and proteins. It's a different story with alcohol. Alcohol is a toxic and foreign substance to the liver. When excessive amounts of alcohol are metabolized, large amounts of hydrogen are built up and retained in the liver. This excess hydrogen is associated with an accumulation of increased fat in the liver. The way this occurs is as follows. The increase in hydrogen inhibits certain metabolic functions in the production of energy; alcohol becomes "preferred fuel," and instead of burning fat the liver burns alcohol. This results in a heavy deposit of fat throughout the liver.

The liver disposes of this excessive fat by releasing it into the blood. This explains why consumption of excessive alcohol always results in elevated blood triglycerides and fats. This is one of the reasons excessive drinkers have a greater degree of premature atherosclerosis than non-drinkers.

Below on the left is an illustration of a healthy, normal liver, metabolizing products it was designed to break down. On the right is the liver metabolizing excessive amounts of alcohol and dumping triglycerides and fats into the blood. Premature atherosclerosis is evident on the artery walls.

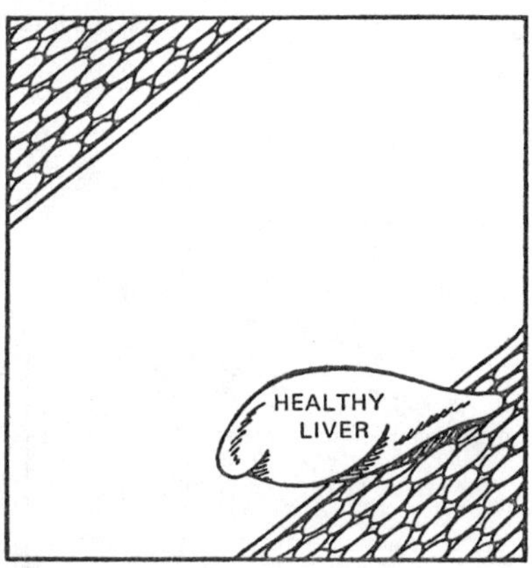

Healthy liver: It is not metabolizing alcohol, and so no triglycerides or fats are being moved into the blood.

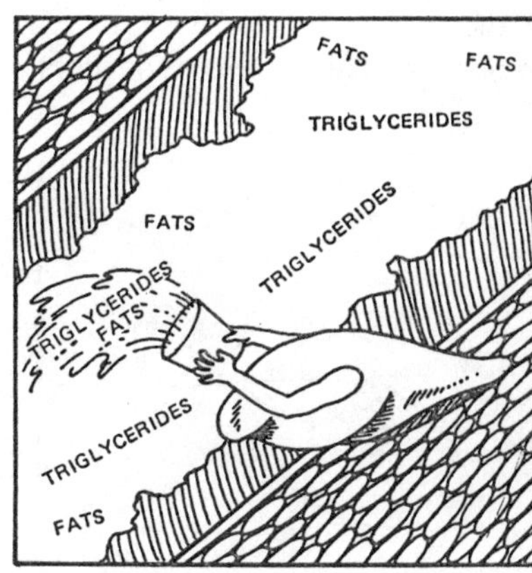

Alcohol stressed liver: Excessive fats and triglycerides in the liver are being dumped into the blood. Note the advanced atherosclerosis.

Early in the course of one's drinking career, this release of fats into the blood is sufficient to keep the liver free from a buildup of fatty tissue. However, with constant and excessive consumption of alcohol, it becomes the prime source of energy metabolism. The accumulation of fat in the liver becomes so great that the liver is not capable of discharging all of it into the blood. This mark of everyday excessive drinking is referred to as "fatty" liver.

Alcohol and the Liver

There are several organs referred to as vital, meaning that without them the body dies. The liver, along with the brain and heart, is particularly vital because, unlike the lungs and kidneys, you have only one. When all liver function stops, the body quickly dies from the buildup of toxic materials which cannot be metabolized. For this reason, any potential problems with the liver are very serious.

As indicated, regular excessive consumption of alcohol causes fatty liver. In this condition, the fat deposits in the liver are the first mark on the liver caused by excess alcohol. Usually the fatty deposits collect into one or more lesions (sores), and the liver becomes soft and flabby and may become enlarged in size.

In the following diagrams, you can see on the left a healthy, normally functioning liver, not required to metabolize everyday doses of alcohol. On the right is a fatty liver, large, soft, and flabby. Pockets of fat tissue can be seen. This liver cannot function to full capacity.

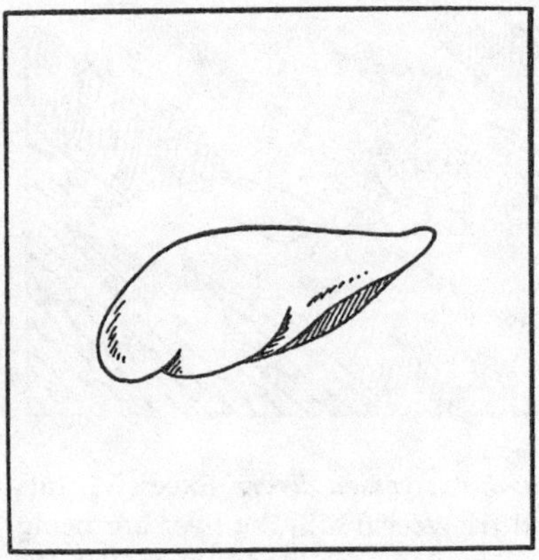

A normal liver: It is capable of a lifetime of metabolic activity.

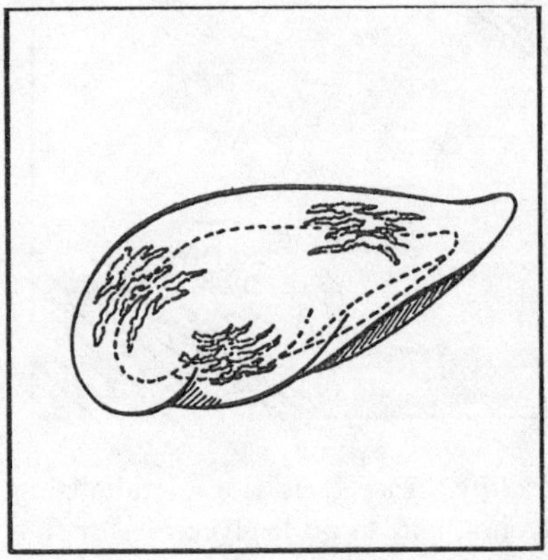

A fatty liver: Fat deposits have become pronounced. The liver is large, soft, and flabby and has lost some of its efficiency.

Hepatitis is an inflammatory disease of the liver which may or may not be associated with a fatty liver. Usually hepatitis is seen only after years of excessive drinking of alcohol. It causes a rise in white cell count, abdominal pain, and jaundice. Hepatitis may advance to cirrhosis of the liver.

Liver cirrhosis usually occurs only after years of alcohol abuse. With the passing of time and the constant demand alcohol metabolism places on the liver, the fatty deposits convert to scar and fiber tissue. When this occurs, the liver decreases in size and becomes tough and leather-like.

Illustrated in the following diagrams are a fatty liver (on the left) and a liver with cirrhosis (on the right) in which the fat tissue has become converted to scar tissue, with the liver function diminished. Studies point out that liver cirrhosis is directly related to the per capita consumption of alcohol. Ten percent of the individuals who consume excessive amounts of alcohol on a regular basis develop liver cirrhosis. Death can result. The actual cause of death is usually rupture of one of the large blood vessels of the liver or cancer of the liver.

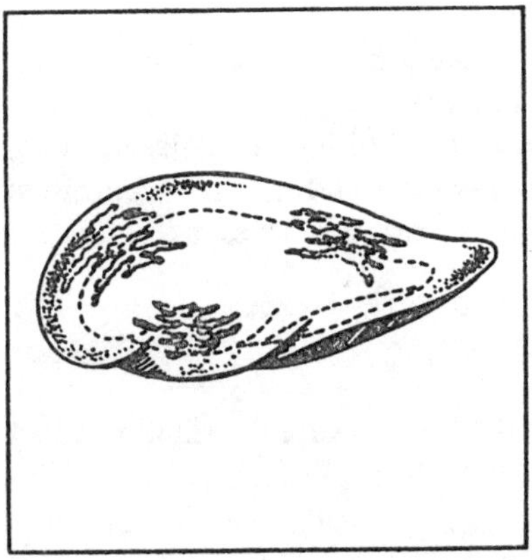

Fatty liver: The result of daily and excessive alcohol consumption.

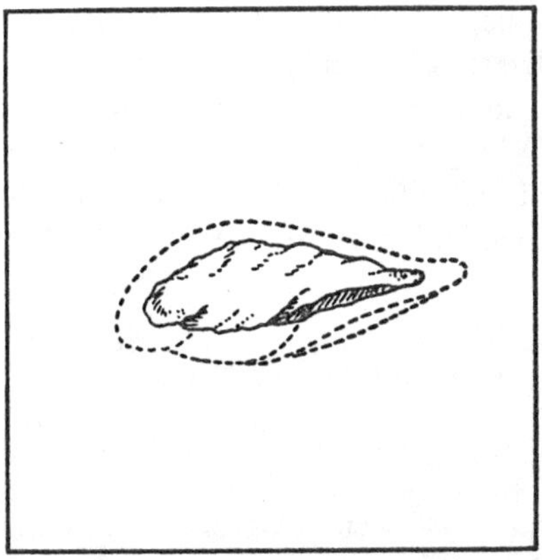

Cirrhosis of the liver: Fatty deposits convert to fiber and scar tissue and the liver shrinks in size. The liver function is reduced.

While permanent damage due to fatty liver, hepatitis, and liver cirrhosis are usually associated with long-term and excessive use of alcohol, liver changes are seen on a temporary basis following alcohol ingestion for short periods of time.

Louise Burgess in her book, *Alcohol and Your Health,* says, "In fact, an increase in liver fat and damage to liver cells were consistently produced after heavy alcohol ingestion for as little as two days." She continues, "Liver injury was produced also by amounts of alcohol that did not cause intoxication, such as are commonly consumed by many so-called social drinkers. This is consistent with the pattern of many individuals who drink considerably in the course of their work and social relationships but who are rarely drunk and who are not considered to be alcoholic persons by their associates. Such individuals, if they consume sufficient alcoholic beverages, appear to increase their susceptibility to liver injury."

As can be seen, alcohol is a toxic material to the liver. The liver does the job requested—metabolizing alcohol—but the price to be paid in liver damage is well understood and documented. As you seek high-level wellness, you must develop your visualization program so as to picture each drink of alcohol causing a buildup in the liver of fat and triglycerides, which are then discharged into your blood. Develop the image of your elevated blood fats and how they contribute to premature atherosclerosis.

Visualize how excessive alcohol causes fat deposits in the liver and what it looks like as it becomes enlarged and flabby. With the passing of time, picture how the fatty tissue converts to scar and fiber tissue and the liver shrinks in size and becomes like leather. Be able to vividly recall what a lifetime of excess alcohol does to the liver.

As you eliminate or limit consumption of alcohol in your daily lifestyle, visualize how each of these conditions is reversed and the liver returns to functioning at full capacity. Get the picture of your liver as a healthy organ.

Alcohol and the Heart

Long-term, excessive alcohol consumption can have a devastating effect on the heart. Studies have pointed out that physical changes occur with fat tissue accumulation in the heart muscle. The heart becomes larger and flabby. In individuals who have seriously abused themselves with alcohol for many years, it is not unusual for the heart to be double normal size. With this degeneration of the heart, there is a decrease in mechanical efficiency.

When the pumping ability of the heart falls below normal, congestive heart failure occurs. In this condition, fluid begins to collect in the lungs and lower extremities of the body. As blood accumulates in the lungs, pulmonary congestion occurs and shortness of breath develops. In other parts of the body, as fluid seeps through capillary walls, edema or swelling occurs, especially in the legs and ankles.

On page 187 are illustrations of the normal heart and a heart that has been exposed to excessive amounts of alcohol for long periods of time.

On the left is a healthy heart, exposed to no or small and infrequent amounts of alcohol. On the right is an alcohol-diseased heart which is larger, flabby, and inefficient.

In addition to congestive heart failure, excessive consumption of alcohol is also involved with an increase in diastolic blood pressure.

When conducting Wellness Seminars, I am often asked about studies

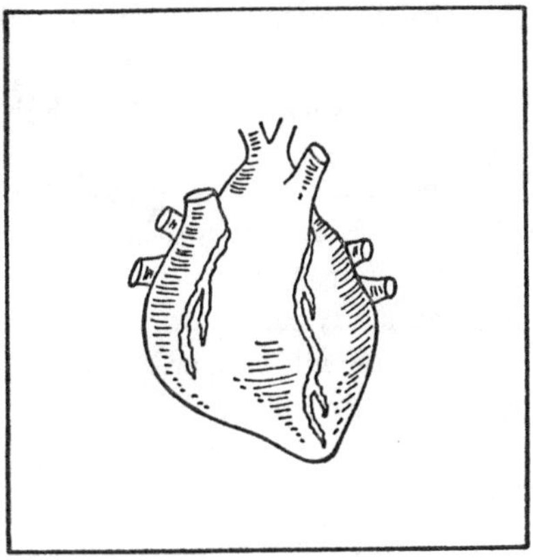

A healthy heart: It is alcohol-free and pumping blood throughout the body with maximum efficiency.

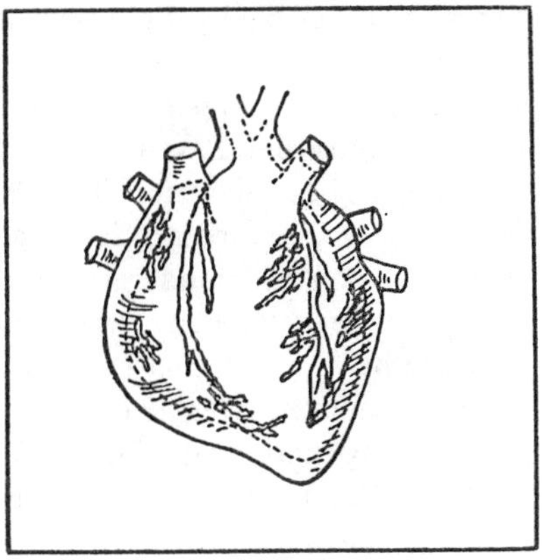

An alcohol-damaged heart: Fat deposits accumulate in the heart muscle and cause a reduction in efficiency. The heart is soft and flabby and may have increased in size.

which received considerable attention recently suggesting that alcohol is beneficial in preventing heart attacks. I have heard the question so often that I would like to answer it here.

Several studies have suggested that modest amounts of alcohol might be beneficial to the heart. It was pointed out that when alcohol blood levels in male volunteers were around 0.05 percent or less, there was an increase in blood flow to the heart muscle. However, when the amount of alcohol was doubled, there was a marked reduction in the velocity of the blood leaving the left side of the heart. This is more proof that excessive consumption of alcohol reduces the efficiency of heart function and is a strong indictment against excessive consumption of alcohol.

A study at Cleveland Clinic pointed out that alcohol causes an increase in HDL levels. HDL is the lipoprotein that collects cholesterol in the blood and returns it to the liver, where it is destroyed. (See chapter 6 for more on HDL and LDL.) On the surface this looks good; however, from a quantitative point of view there is no reason to look to alcohol as a cure for heart diseases. It was found that when two drinks are consumed each day there is an increase in HDL of 6 percent. This is not statistically significant and is therefore meaningless. In addition there was a rise in LDL. LDL picks up cholesterol and distributes it throughout the body. It was necessary for the subjects to drink four or more drinks per day in order to get a 15 percent increase (statistically significant) in HDL with no appreciable rise in LDL.

Another study is from the Oakland Kaiser-Permanente Medical Center.

Over eight thousand people were divided in four groups: teetotalers, moderate drinkers (two or less drinks per day), moderate to heavy drinkers (three to five drinks per day), and heavy drinkers (six or more drinks per day). They were followed for ten years.

This study is interesting because it uses death as an end point. They found the highest death rate occurred among the heavy drinkers and lowest among the moderate drinkers (lower than for the teetotalers). Many will be watching and waiting to see if this study can be duplicated.

It can be expected that more studies of this type will appear. I offer one word of caution. Even if it is eventually proved that alcohol is beneficial in reducing cardiovascular diseases, the documented and understood harmful effects must always be considered.

What you must do is learn to visualize exactly how excessive alcohol causes an increase in fat tissue within the heart muscle and causes it to become enlarged, flabby, and inefficient. Picture the oversized, lazy heart allowing fluid and blood to accumulate in your lungs and throughout the body. Get the feeling of the overall effect this tired, struggling heart has on blood circulation.

As you eliminate or limit alcohol consumption, visualize the heart returning to normal size and becoming stronger. With proper visualization, your alcohol consumption can be modified.

Alcohol and the Gastrointestinal Tract

Any quantity of alcohol stimulates gastric acid production. With larger quantities of alcohol, the gastric mucosal barrier (protective coating of the stomach) is damaged. This results in an increase in the possibility of gastric ulcers.

Alcohol seems to impair absorption from the small intestine. Studies have pointed out that when well-fed volunteers are given large amounts of alcohol, absorption of amino acids, vitamins, fats, and sugars was reduced. From this it can be concluded that alcohol can hinder the function of the ileum (small intestine) even when nutrition is adequate.

Long-term, excessive alcohol consumption can cause problems with the pancreas. The pancreas is the organ that secretes insulin, which is involved in controlling blood sugar levels. In addition, digestive enzymes are produced. The pancreas usually responds to alcohol overdose with general inflammation and a reduction in overall pancreas activity.

Alcohol and Cancer

There is no doubt that alcohol causes cancer, and its consumption is one of the types of exposure definitely proved to increase the risk of cancer at various sites in the body. In comparison to the general population, individuals who consume excessive alcohol *always* have a higher incidence of cancer of the mouth and pharynx, larynx (throat), esophagus, liver, and stomach.

Alcohol consumption in combination with smoking increases the risk for developing cancer of the upper respiratory tract and the digestive tract. One theory advanced to explain this observation is that tobacco carcinogens might more easily gain access to the mucous membrane if the cells are bathed in alcohol.

Cancer of the esophagus, which is the tube from the mouth to the stomach, is influenced by alcohol more than any other. Consumption of excessive amounts of hard liquor seems to cause cancer more frequently than consumption of excessive amounts of beer or wine. When individuals smoke and drink, the chance for cancer of the esophagus is further increased. Studies have proved that there is a relationship between the amount of alcohol consumed and cigarettes smoked and the incidence of cancer. The greater the amount of alcohol and number of cigarettes, the more frequent the cancer.

Below are several illustrations showing how and why cancer of the mouth and pharynx, larynx, and esophagus is more frequent in those who consume excess alcohol.

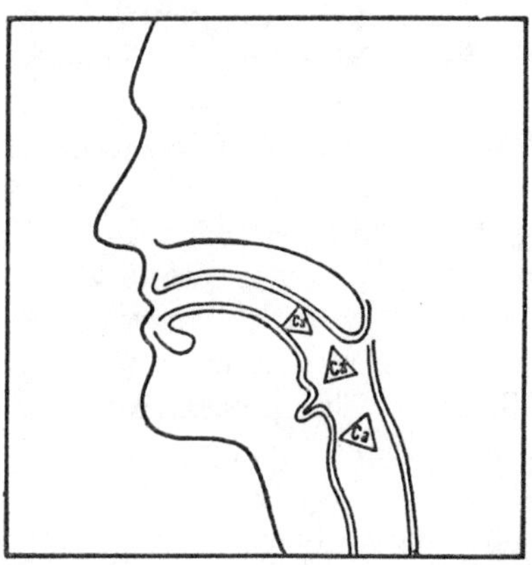

Natural protective coating: A barrier normally coats the mouth, throat, and esophagus and protects them from cancer-causing toxins.

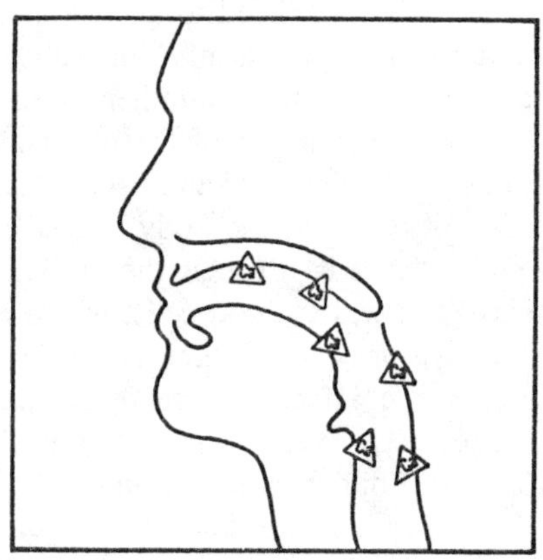

Depleted coating: Regular alcohol ingestion removes the protective coating and makes it easier for cancer toxins to invade.

On the left can be seen the protective coating of the oral cavity, throat, and esophagus, which may prevent the invasion of cancer-causing agents. On the right, the protective coating is removed because of drinking regular and excessive amounts of alcohol. Under this condition, the cancer toxins have better access to the tissue where cancer can start.

Excessive consumption of alcohol has been associated with cancer of the liver and the stomach. Studies have pointed out that alcohol alone will cause liver cancer. Stomach cancer may be due to agents in the alcoholic drink other than alcohol itself. All alcoholic beverages contain chemicals in addition to ethyl alcohol. Carcinogenic agents have been found in many alcoholic beverages. Beer, wine, vermouth, and sherry have been found to contain asbestos fibers. Other contaminants found in alcoholic beverages are polycyclic hydrocarbons and benzene compounds.

In summary, alcohol alone or in combination with smoking causes an increase in cancer of the oral cavity, throat, and esophagus. You must develop the ability to visualize excessive alcohol removing the protective barrier from the mouth, throat, esophagus, and stomach. Picture carcinogens being able to attack the unprotected tissue lining these parts of the body. As you eliminate or reduce alcohol consumption, visualize a tough protective coating, one which carcinogens cannot penetrate. Picture yourself with the reduced possibility of cancer of the mouth, throat, esophagus, and stomach.

Alcohol and Infections

The body is exposed to and, in fact, contains bacteria at all times. Some of the bacteria are harmful and others have beneficial functions. The body can tolerate a certain number of the harmful bacteria with no problem, but when the number of these organisms reaches a certain elevated level, you develop symptoms and become sick.

One of the ways the body keeps the number of bacteria down to an acceptable level is through the activities of the lymphocytes (white blood cells). The white blood cells, which are produced by the lymph system of the body, move to the area of the body where there are too many bacteria (site of the infection), surround and kill them. This process is called phagocytosis. This system works well and will keep a healthy person free from infections most of the time.

Excessive consumption of alcohol prohibits the movement of the white blood cells. When this occurs, the body has lost all or a portion of its ability to fight infections. On page 191, to the left, is an illustration of how the white cells keep the bacteria under control. They surround the bacteria, kill them, and move them out of the body. On the right is what happens in the case of excessive consumption of alcohol. The white cells cannot move to the site of bacteria buildup and, therefore, the bacteria are free to reproduce and spread. As the number of bacteria increases, symptoms become more severe.

In the case of serious alcohol abuse, infections such as pneumonia are very common. This is caused by the inability of white cells to migrate to the site of the infection. Under these conditions, it is not unusual for the

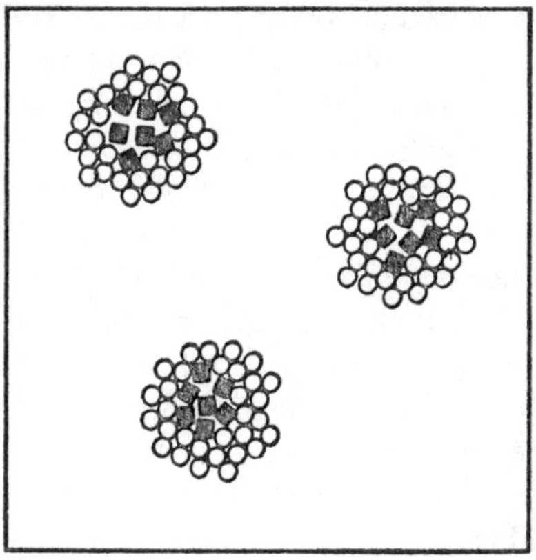

Phagocytosis: White blood cells surround bacteria and prevent their spread and reproduction.

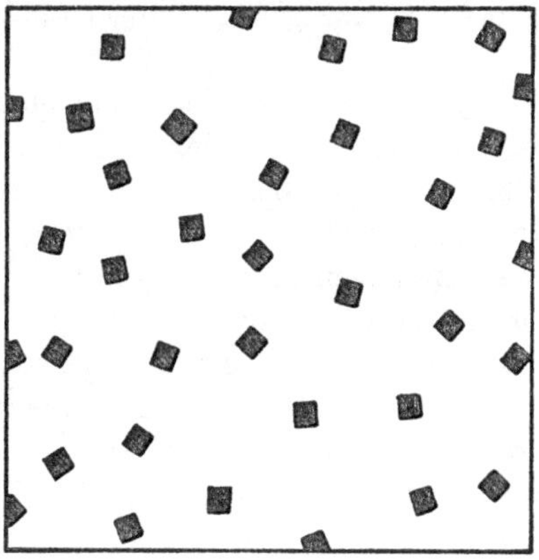

Alcohol and infection: Alcohol inhibits the movement of white blood cells and bacteria spread and reproduce in an uncontrolled way.

individual to experience frequent problems with sinusitis, bronchitis, pharyngitis, and deep chest colds.

Develop your own ability to learn about and visualize how excessive alcohol prohibits white cell migration and impedes the body's defense system against bacterial reproduction and infections. As you begin to limit or eliminate alcohol consumption, picture your white cells getting free, traveling to the site of the infection. Visualize your vibrant white cells rushing to that part of your body where the bacteria count is starting to increase. Think of your white cells surrounding the bacteria and killing them by strangulation. Visualize yourself as infection-free, feeling good, and achieving high-level wellness.

HOW TO ELIMINATE OR REDUCE ALCOHOL CONSUMPTION

By now, you have some idea of how and why excessive alcohol destroys vital organs and body systems. You have also had the opportunity to study a number of illustrations that allow you to visualize the impact excess alcohol has, and the changes that will occur as you eliminate or reduce your alcohol consumption.

There is a close association between consumption of excess alcohol and the lack of high-level wellness. It is impossible to experience any degree of wellness in the face of excess alcohol. Alcohol alters mind function and has a devastating impact on vital organs and body systems. If you want to assure the highest level of wellness, eliminate alcohol from your lifestyle. If you find this is absolutely impossible, limit your consumption of alcohol along the lines suggested in this chapter. Remember, alcohol is a foreign and toxic drug. High-level wellness and excessive alcohol cannot reside in the same body.

If you haven't already, you must now decide if your goal is to eliminate or reduce your consumption of alcohol. If it's elimination, that's good. If it's reduction, you should have a well-defined upper limit on your daily consumption. The experts agree that the absolute maximum is three cocktails or beers or glasses of wine per twenty-four-hour period. Your goal may be this or anything less. In addition, you must plan your drinking so there are periods when you drink nothing so as to give the liver a rest from metabolizing alcohol. This can be two days per week or one week per month.

Step One: *Make your personal commitment to reduce or eliminate alcohol consumption.* By now you have decided that your goal is either to reduce your consumption of alcohol or to eliminate it completely. It doesn't matter which is your goal, the approach is the same.

You must make your personal commitment. The way you do this is to carefully think through and answer this question: "Why is the reduction or elimination of alcohol from my lifestyle so important to me?" Do not move forward with your program until you have the answer. The next question you must ask is, "How important is it for me to achieve this goal?" Try to place a priority on this project as compared to other activities in your life. You must become convinced of the importance of reducing or eliminating alcohol.

After you have the answers, I want you to write a brief summary. Your summary can be as short or long as you wish. The important thing is for you to have thoroughly analyzed your situation instead of blindly, without forethought, starting your program. By writing down the answers you have discovered, you are providing information for your mind about how and why reduction or elimination of alcohol is important to you.

Avoid the temptation to think about or concentrate on other negative lifestyles. Many people make the mistake of thinking they can control the mind and place equal emphasis on the elimination of more than one negative lifestyle. It can't be done. If you dilute your educational and visualization program, the result will be failure.

Your mind must take over and readjust your body regulators so that excessive alcohol is no longer an okay activity and, therefore, is rejected. In order to do this, you must place complete and undiluted effort behind a single project. The mind will always respond with proper body signals if the goal is clear and singular concentration given.

Step Two: *Study and review the material and illustrations in this book which explain how and why excessive alcohol destroys vital organs and body systems.* The reason you presently consume more alcohol than you want to is because you do not fully comprehend how and why excessive alcohol is harmful. Once you have adequate information, convert it into personal knowledge. You will then have the foundation to build your program of wellness self-responsibility.

As you study the material, understand how excess alcohol causes red blood cell sludging and how this kills untold brain cells by blocking capillary blood flow. Learn how the liver metabolizes alcohol, causing hydrogen collection in the liver, and how the hydrogen causes an increase of fat in the liver. Know how this excess fat is dumped into the blood, increasing the levels of triglycerides and other fats. Understand that with continued exposure to excess alcohol, the liver cannot discharge all the fat it collects, and this results in a fatty liver. Comprehend how a fatty liver may become associated with hepatitis and cirrhosis. Learn how excess alcohol causes fat accumulation in the heart muscle and how its efficiency is dramatically decreased. Learn how alcohol is a caustic to the stomach and intestines. Understand the role of excessive alcohol in causing cancer of the mouth, throat, and esophagus. Understand how and why excess alcohol is involved in inhibiting the body's ability to fight infections.

Learn the details as to why and how these things happen. Know how alcohol provides an inebriated feeling by anesthetizing portions of the brain. Know how the body responds to various concentrations of alcohol in the blood. Learn about the upper limits of normal for safe alcohol consumption.

You may wish to have information beyond that provided in this book. That's fine. Your library or Alcoholics Anonymous will be pleased to provide you with additional information. Become your own private expert on the overall effects of excessive alcohol on the mind and body.

Step Three: *Develop the ability to mentally visualize how excess alcohol destroys your vital organs and body systems.* Numerous illustrations are provided in this chapter. As you are studying the material, also study the illustrations. Get them fixed in your mind and know what they mean. First, be able to mentally recall the illustration that shows the effect excessive alcohol has in harming your vital organs and body systems. Since your mind is not yet filled with information about the harmful effects of excessive alcohol, the illustrations along with the information provided are used to give the mind a picture of what is now occurring to your vital organs and body systems.

Next, use the illustration of the normal organ and body function to show the mind what you want to achieve. It is important to always provide this mental visual goal. The mind will always respond with appropriate body signals if the instructions are clear.

By using these "before and after" mental pictures, the mind becomes convinced that excess alcohol is harmful and generates signals to the body that excess alcohol is not to be tolerated. At this time, the desire for alcohol no longer exists, or exists only up to certain limits.

Step Four: *Write a detailed summary of everything you learn about how and why excessive alcohol destroys vital organs and body systems.* As you are learning about the harmful effects of excess alcohol, take notes. You will have a much better recall if you write as you learn. Numerous studies have proved that learning is faster and retained longer if the material is written.

After you have completed your study program, use your notes to write a detailed summary about how and why excessive alcohol is harmful. Your written summary is a controlled and disciplined way for you to be sure that all the material has been covered and allows you to become actively involved in educating your mind.

As you are doing your written summary, you should also experiment with creating your own visualization illustrations. As you are turning over in your mind your new information about the harm alcohol does to you, think about what it looks like. Convert knowledge into your own mental pictures. Then turn the mental pictures into drawings. Anatomical correctness is not important. What is important is your involvement and for you to have as many vehicles as possible to communicate to your mind pictures of the harmful effects, and of what changes will take place as alcohol is eliminated or curtailed. Use the illustrations in this chapter as a guide but feel free to supplement them with your own. Visualization illustrations that you create will be more meaningful to you than any I can provide.

Step Five: *Practice your visualization program every morning upon waking, and at midday, evening, bedtime, and any time there is an urge to drink.* Getting started on your program of visualization will initially require discipline on your part. You must have a fixed and definite schedule so that visualization will become a part of your daily routine. At first, effort is required to establish your schedule, but soon visualization will become a habit.

You should conduct your first visualization session as soon as you wake in the morning. While lying in bed, run through your mental television illustrations of all the harmful effects of excess alcohol. See them clearly. Tell your mind that this is what excess alcohol does. Next, visualize how your vital organs and body systems will look after you have eliminated or reduced your consumption of alcohol. Tell your mind that this is what you want to accomplish.

This same visual program should be conducted midmorning, around lunch, midafternoon, and around dinnertime. It is obvious you must have adequate time for your visualization and the time must be uninterrupted.

The best time for visualization is just before going to sleep. The mind functions during sleep and can be instructed and taught at this time. Some think that this is ideal because there are no distractions. After you are relaxed in bed, run your entire program through your mind. By visualizing just before going to sleep and upon awakening, the mind is given a constant twenty-four-hour base for education.

You should visualize each time you have the urge to drink or are actually drinking. This activity will make you aware of how much and what you are drinking. By using visualization at this time, you will be amazed how often you can refuse that first drink or stop after one or two.

Step Six: *Determine and write down a schedule or target date whereby you either will eliminate alcohol or will be at or below your goal.* One of the most important steps of your program is to establish a specific schedule or date for the accomplishment of definite predetermined goals.

If you have decided to eliminate alcohol completely, you may wish to stop abruptly or to reduce down to zero according to a schedule. If it's the former, select the day when you will stop. If you are going to reduce down to no alcohol, establish a definite maximum number of drinks per day, and reduce it each week. For example, if you are now having three or four drinks every day, you might have a goal of a maximum of three per day this week, then two per day the following week, then one per day the third week. Establish the last day of the third week as the last day you will ever consume alcohol.

If your objective is to limit your consumption of alcohol, determine what your daily maximum is going to be. Remember, three drinks per day is maximum with forty-eight hours each week or one week each month in which there is no alcohol. Most people find with the passing of time that they continue to reduce the upper limit of drinks they consume.

It is vital that your goals be written down. When you establish a definite goal, you give the mind a target. When you write down the goal, you are informing the mind you are serious and expect prompt response in the form of new signals being sent to the body for the limitation or elimination of alcohol.

Step Seven: *Develop a vivid mental image of you consuming either no alcohol or limited amounts of alcohol.* Picture yourself today as the end product you want to be. Visualize yourself either without alcohol in your life or in a reduced amount. Think about the difference between you without a hangover and all those who have one. Visualize how great you will look and feel without the cobwebs of alcohol in your brain. Get a picture of, and actually feel, how good it will be without alcohol. Drinking is expensive. Calculate how much you will save by eliminating or reducing your drinking. Figure out in advance what you will buy with the extra income. Picture in advance all the advantages you will realize from eliminating excessive alcohol from your lifestyle.

This approach to the elimination or reduction of alcohol consumption will work for you. The reason I can be so sure is because after you have conditioned your mind, you really have no control. Your mind will not tolerate any abuse of the body which it understands to be harmful. You have at your disposal everything required for you to know HOW TO MODERATE YOUR DRINKING—OR QUIT COMPLETELY IF YOU WISH.

ADDITIONAL HELPFUL HINTS

At the end of each chapter you are provided with a brief outline of practical information, tips, and hints that are intended to supplement your visualization program. When used in conjunction with visualization, they will help you eliminate your negative lifestyle.

These practical hints to help you eliminate or reduce alcohol consumption provide a number of suggestions that will assist you in achieving your goal.

1) Ask yourself, "Why am I having this drink, beer, or glass of wine?" Is it out of habit? To relax? To forget what happened today? To become intoxicated? The reason doesn't matter. Get into the habit of asking yourself this question every time you drink. Often you will find the answer is, "I don't know." In many cases the next step is to say, "I don't think I will have this drink after all."

2) Set a definite schedule for no drinking. You may begin by not drinking on Monday, Wednesday, and Thursday. Then expand your no-drinking to Monday through Friday. The age-old rule of no drinking before five o'clock is good.

3) Place a limit on the number of cocktails, beers, or wine you have each day.

4) Many people drink out of habit. They drink at a certain time or because of a particular happening. If you are in the habit of "popping a top" or mixing a drink as soon as you arrive home, always have a large glass of fruit juice first. You will be surprised how often the juice alone will satisfy you.

5) When you develop the urge for a drink, *EXERCISE*. Go for a walk, vacuum the house, ride the bike. Divert your attention away from having a drink and get away from the place where the alcohol is stored. This is the best of all substitutes for drinking.

6) Make it difficult to drink at home. Keep the beer in the basement. Store the liquor in that part of the house most distant from where you mix drinks.

7) If you have never tried it, say, "No, thanks," when offered a drink. Many have found, in this day and age, that it commands more respect than saying yes.

8) Try your favorite drink without alcohol. If you regularly drink Bloody Marys, try the mix complete with lime and celery stalk. It may surprise you that going through the mechanics and having a glass to sip from will satisfy you.

9) Always order or mix your drinks in a tall glass. While the extra mixer (except water) does provide additional calories, the alcohol is diluted more.

10) When you order a mixed drink, ask for an extra side glass of mixer. As you sip the drink, refill your glass with the mixer. This can cut your alcohol consumption in half.

11) If you are a beer drinker, try it in a tall glass filled with ice. Not only does it make the beer colder, but sipping from an ice-filled glass is slower than gulping from a can or bottle.

12) At home, experiment with various fruit juices instead of the six o'clock cocktail. Cranberry juice is different and satisfying.

13) When you have a cocktail, beer, or wine, sip it *very* slowly.

14) Drinking is expensive. As you reduce alcohol consumption or eliminate it completely, keep a record of the large amount of money you are saving.

15) Establish a reward system for yourself. Save the money accumulated by reduction or elimination of alcohol for three months. You will be surprised how much it is. Go out and spend all of it on yourself. Buy something you have wanted but didn't think you could afford.

16) Resolve that you will *never* become drunk again.

17) Make a rule that you will not drive if you have had more than two drinks.

9. PHYSICAL FITNESS TODAY, TOMORROW, AND FOREVER

"That which is used develops,
that which is not used wastes away."
HIPPOCRATES

I started on a program of regular exercise about nine years ago. At that time I started running. During the past nine years I cannot recall a span of more than three days with no running. I average running six days a week in spite of an extensive travel schedule.

I can remember vividly when I started this habit which has been with me for so long. I was on a business trip and had stopped in Puerto Rico on the way to South America. I was staying on the ocean in the Dorado Beach area. It was on a weekend, so business activities were minimal. The beach in front of the hotel is one of the most beautiful in the world. On a Saturday morning I decided to take a walk on the beach. As I was walking along, taking in the rugged beauty of the coast, I decided I would run to a cove about two hundred yards ahead. I started off at a very slow trot. I made it to the cove without stopping, but I was completely out of breath and exhausted. I suppose it was at that moment that it dawned on me how deconditioned I was. I had never taken time to reflect on the state of my personal physical condition. I decided that Saturday morning that I would run the next morning. On Sunday I made the decision to run on Monday.

After the decision was made to try to run every day, I began concentrating on the distance. I must tell you that by today's standards my progress was slow. It took me about two months to work up to a mile a day. I thought that was great! I was doing something few people could do—run a mile.

All of us who are running today know a mile is not even a good warm-up, but you must consider the conditions nine years ago. Running was not an "in" thing to do. There were no sophisticated running shoes—I used a flat-soled pair of sneakers. Elaborate warm-up and running clothes did not exist—my warm-up was a pair of old baggy gray sweat pants with elastic around the ankles. When I ran in the neighborhood everyone was saying, "What's wrong with him, is he crazy?" Nine years ago the Boston Marathon, the New York Marathon, the Peachtree Roadrace, the Vulcan Run either did not exist or were run by only a fraction of the thousands who now run each year.

What a difference nine years makes. Figures are not available to estimate the number of people who were running on a regular basis then, but today we know that over 25 million men, women, and children are running on a regular basis. Today, entries in excess of 10,000 are not uncommon at the popular marathon races, with thousands turned away. Thousands of 10,000-meter races are run throughout the nation in cities large and small. There are large retail stores that specialize exclusively in running equipment. Now there are dozens of brands, models, and colors of running shoes. The wearing apparel on the track is a cause of extreme consideration to the discriminating runner. In the early days, running seemed to be primarily a man's activity. Not now. Women have not only moved onto the track, but they compete with equal zest and conditioning.

The point is that several years ago most people said running was a fad. It's something people would do for six months, a year, at most two years, and then get tired of it. Time has proved these prognosticators wrong! Running is here to stay and growing every day.

With all this consideration of running, you might get the impression that this chapter is devoted only to this subject. Not true. This chapter is on the subject of total physical fitness—how to start on a program of regular exercise and stay on it so that physical fitness will become a reality.

Valid statistics are available that show large numbers of people are exercising on a regular basis. The so-called "exercise craze" started in the early or mid-1970s. Prior to that time the numbers who exercised on a regular basis were few. Today, based on figures from the National Center for Health Statistics, it is estimated that the following are involved in these exercises on a regular basis (some are involved in more than one exercise):

Numbers Who Exercise Regularly

46 million walk
30 million play tennis
25 million run or jog
25 million play squash-racquet-handball

22 million bowl
18 million do calisthenics
15 million ride a bicycle
12 million play golf

When one first looks at these figures they seem impressive. From the standpoint of improvement made from 1970 until 1980 they *are* impressive, but what must also be considered are the percentages of the total population engaged in these exercises.

It is estimated that about 18 percent of the population walk as a form of regular exercise. About 12 percent play tennis. Ten percent run or jog, and an equal number play one of the racquetball court games. Approximately 9 percent bowl and 7 percent do calisthenics on a daily basis. Six percent ride a bicycle and about 5 percent play golf.

So, even though the number of people now involved in regular exercise is high, many times that of five or ten years ago, the total percentage of those exercising is low. I point this out so that it can clearly be seen that even though progress has been made, much still needs to be done in order to double or triple the percentage of Americans involved in regular exercise.

The question should be raised why such a low percentage of Americans are involved in an exercise program. The answer is simple. Starting on a program of regular exercise is easy. Becoming conditioned so as to continue the program is difficult. People can get excited about starting an exercise program because in this country almost everyone is fairly active in grade and high school. Even into college, through physical education classes and intramural programs, individuals maintain a certain level of physical fitness. Because of this regular exercise in early life, most know about and appreciate the value of physical fitness. So, all you have to do for many people is simply suggest that they start to become involved in a program for regular exercise and a large percentage will say, "When do I start?" *The problem is that 68 percent of those who are motivated to start a program of regular exercise are no longer exercising at the end of thirty days.*

Why is it that so many people who start down the road to high-level physical fitness run out of gas? Why is the failure rate so high? Have you ever started on a new program for regular exercise and for some reason fallen back into the old habits of the sedentary life? If you are like most, the answer is yes. At the present time a war is being waged within your body. On one side are the millions of cells of your body which are on the search for more oxygen. On the other side are your deconditioned heart and lungs which have grown lazy and inefficient through lack of exertion. You must become involved in this war. You must do battle against a life that lacks energy, enthusiasm, optimism, pride, and self-satisfaction.

I recently read: "In the United States, from a physical fitness point of view, most people are middle-aged by the time they are 26 and old at 34." How incredibly sad, but true. Do you question the validity of this observation? If so, ask the average person who does not exercise to run up three flights of stairs. Ask them to run the length of a football field. Ask them to swim four laps in the YMCA pool. Ask them to play one fast game of racquetball. More than likely they can't. If they do, they will be breathing so hard they can hardly talk.

PREMATURE AGING

We are now living in the age when everyone wants to stay young and attractive forever. If you doubt this for one moment, check with your local plastic surgeon. Twenty or thirty years ago cosmetic surgery (face-lifts, hair transplants, and breast reconstruction) was rarely done outside the entertainment field. Now you are hardpressed to get an appointment with a good plastic surgeon. Thousands of people are trying to pursue youth and attractiveness with a knife.

The problem with these procedures is that they do nothing to alter the aging process. One activity which will slow down the aging process is regular, sustained exercise and physical fitness. Now I am not suggesting that physical fitness will grow hair, but I am suggesting you have two choices. One is the life you are now living, one in which the cells of your body are being deprived of the oxygen necessary for reproduction and maintenance. The other is the life of physical fitness and a highly conditioned body where there is more than adequate oxygen for cell reproduction, which will put the brake on the aging process.

The President's Council on Physical Fitness and Sports has said:

> Regular exercise primes the immune system (the cells and antibodies that protect us against disease) and helps our brain and body resist aging. If human brain and body are kept in good condition, they deteriorate less rapidly.

If you want to slow down the aging process, if you want to minimize your chances for premature death, come along with me. I am going to share with you a plan that will get you started on your program for physical fitness and that will result in high-level wellness you never thought possible. But more important, with this plan you will still be on your program for top-notch conditioning one year from now, ten years from now, for as long as you live. If you play golf, you will enjoy walking; you will walk or ride your bike to the grocery store; you will stay away from the escalator and elevators and you won't even mind pushing the lawn mower. Because of this program you truly will feel better and live longer.

THE DECONDITIONED BODY

The first step in learning how to start and remain on a program of regular, sustained exercise is to have a good working knowledge of the results of the sedentary life. What are the effects of deconditioning (lack of regular, sustained exercise)?

It is amazing how quickly deconditioning can occur. If a person who is in top physical condition misses regular exercise sessions for one week, deconditioning starts. Can you imagine what occurs in the individual who has not engaged in regular exercise in ten, twenty, perhaps thirty years? Deconditioning affects the entire body and mind.

I want to begin by considering what deconditioning does to the major vital organs and body systems. As indicated in the beginning of this book I want to introduce you to new ways of thinking. I do not want you to think of your body as one huge glob of deconditioned protoplasm. Instead, I want you to think about the vital organs and body systems as separate entities. In other words, I want you to think about your heart as being deconditioned, your lungs as being deconditioned, your blood vessels as being deconditioned, your muscles as being deconditioned, and so forth. After all, the huge glob of protoplasm (you) is the sum total of each of the factors. If you can comprehend the effects of deconditioning at the organ and system level, you will develop a much better understanding of your problem. In addition, you will be able to incorporate your strongest ally—*visualization.*

When we talk about exercising, I want you to be able to mentally visualize each of your vital organs and body systems being individually exercised and understand how and why each responds to the exercise.

The Heart

The heart is the most active muscle in the body. It contracts over one hundred thousand times each day. You might think any muscle this active would be in peak condition. Not so, because this is a minimum work load for the heart. It is doing only as much as it has to do and still get the job done. The heart that is not taken above the customary 72–74 beats per minute for extended periods of time is lazy. It becomes lethargic and, even though it does an adequate job of pumping blood throughout the body, it is not nearly as efficient as it could be.

Any muscle that is not exercised for extended periods of time decreases in size and strength. If you were a high school or college athlete or if you have ever been on a regular calisthenics program, developed good muscle definition, and then stopped the exercise, what happened? The muscle definition disappeared and the muscle mass became smaller. The muscles turned soft and flabby. You will also notice a difference in strength. As long as you exercised the muscle, you experienced an increase in the number of repetitions you could do. If you stopped the calisthenics for a period of time and then started back again, you could not do as many as before. The heart reacts to exercise in exactly the same way.

Now, what happens when the heart is exercised on a regular and sustained basis?

Perhaps we should first stop and reflect on how you go about exercising the heart. The only way to make it work harder is to make it contract faster. This is accomplished by creating an oxygen deficit throughout the body. The oxygen deficit is caused by overall body exercise. Once you have the heart contracting faster due to exercise, it is essential that the elevated rate of contraction be sustained for a period of time. For individuals who are in good condition, this period should be at least twenty and preferably thirty minutes. An important word of caution. It will take you a period of time to get to the point where you can exercise continuously for twenty to thirty minutes. If you are deconditioned, don't overdo it at first. You should consider checking with your physician before starting. Often the question comes up about how often the heart should be exercised. The ideal is every day—at the minimum, every other day.

How vigorous should your heart exercise be? It's based upon Estimated Maximum Heart Rate (EMHR). EMHR is discussed in detail later in this chapter. After your heart is in good condition, you should not exceed 80 percent of your EMHR. So regular exercise means five or six times a week. Sustained exercise means, for the conditioned heart, twenty to thirty minutes—not to exceed 80 percent of EMHR.

Unless you are a part of a surgical team, you have probably never seen a human heart. For this reason, you must envision what the heart looks like based upon drawings or photographs. There are usually physical differences between the deconditioned and the conditioned heart. The deconditioned but normal heart may be slightly smaller in size, and its most important factor cannot be seen: it is weaker than the conditioned heart. The well-conditioned heart may be slightly larger in size and it's stronger and better developed.

What happens as the heart becomes firmer and stronger? It is able to pump a greater volume of blood with each contraction. This conditioning effect is easy to observe.

In the deconditioned person, the resting heart rate will usually be 72 beats or more per minute for men and slightly higher for women. As regular and sustained exercise progresses and the heart becomes stronger, the resting heart rate goes down. Mine is around 52 beats per minute. Stop and take your pulse. What is your resting heart rate? It is a good indication of how conditioned or deconditioned your heart really is. If you are a man and your resting heart rate is 72 or above, your heart is probably deconditioned. For women, if it is 76 or above, you probably have a deconditioned heart. Now you may be wondering why all the fuss just because my heart beats slower than yours. If your resting heart rate is 72, your heart is contracting 28,800 times more often during each twenty-four-hour period than mine.

When you condition your heart, it becomes a more efficient machine. The job of the heart is to push blood throughout the body. Cardiac conditioning causes the blood to be pumped with less effort. Since the conditioned heart is contracting less often, the rest period between contractions is longer. Some are of the opinion that this extra rest has a long-term cumulative and beneficial effect. Others do not subscribe to this conclusion. Following is an artist's conception of what the conditioned and the deconditioned heart might look like.

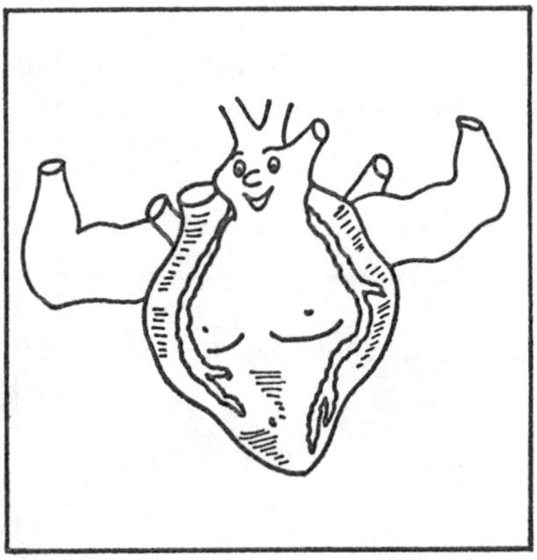

The conditioned heart: It is firm and strong, pumping more blood with each contraction.

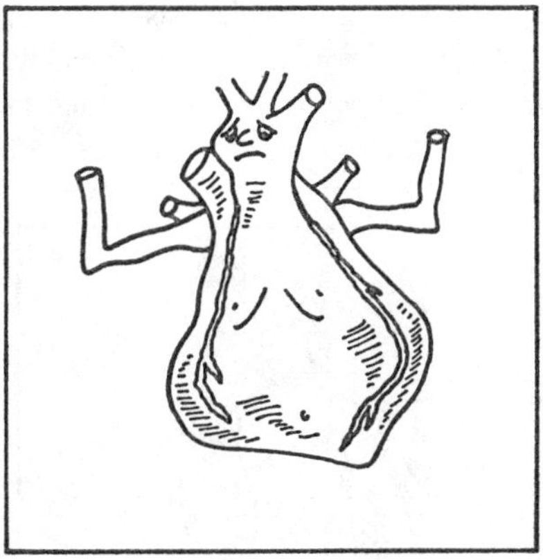

The deconditioned heart: It may be small. It is always soft and lazy. It must labor at full capacity just to circulate the blood.

You must develop the ability to visualize what the deconditioned heart looks like as it goes about its laborious task of pushing the blood throughout your body. On the other hand, picture in your mind the tremendous transformation that will take place as your heart becomes conditioned. Like any other muscle, it firms up. It becomes stronger.

In addition to heart rate, another positive effect of exercise to the heart is increased vascularization. Even though the heart is filled with oxygen-rich blood at all times, this blood is not available to the heart muscle itself. Oxygen-carrying blood is supplied to the heart muscle through the coronary arteries. Studies have pointed out that the coronary arteries become larger in the conditioned heart. In other words, in the conditioned heart, the blood and oxygen supply to the heart muscle is greater. This means more healthy heart muscle.

In the deconditioned heart, not only are the coronary arteries smaller, but atherosclerosis may be more pronounced. Atherosclerosis is the buildup of foreign material on the interior of an artery. The result is a narrowing of the internal diameter of the artery and, therefore, a slowing of blood flow. There is controversy as to whether exercise prevents atherosclerosis, but most do agree that regular, sustained exercise will reduce the incidence of atherosclerosis throughout the circulatory system. Thus, in the deconditioned heart you have a situation in which the coronary arteries are smaller, with reduced blood flow due to atherosclerosis. In the conditioned heart, the coronary arteries become larger and there is less atherosclerosis.

Below are two illustrations which show the difference in cardiac vascularization in the conditioned and the deconditioned heart.

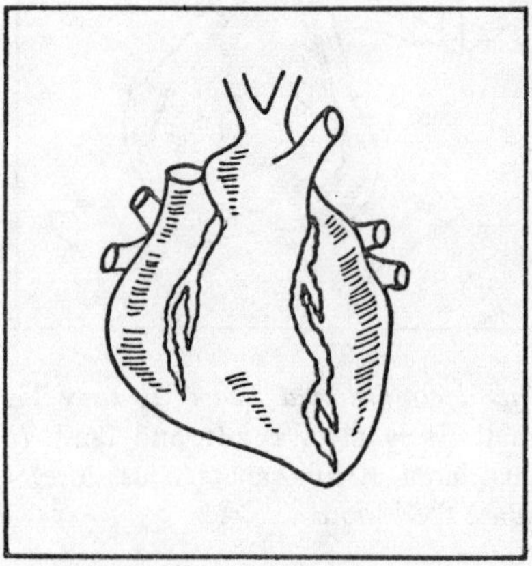

Conditioned coronary circulation: The coronary arteries are like major rivers supplying the heart muscle with more than enough oxygen.

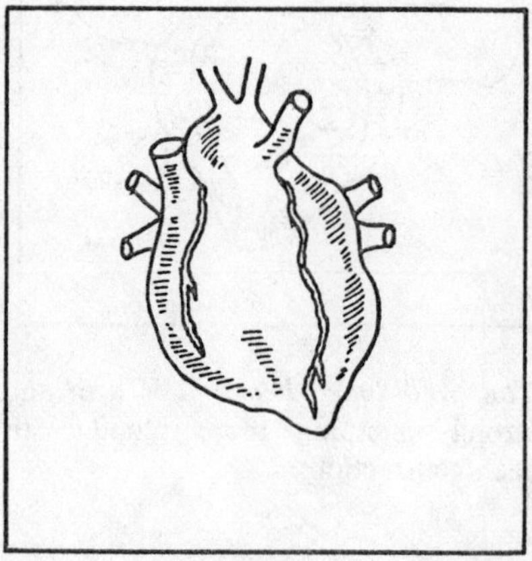

Deconditioned coronary circulation: The coronary arteries are small and may be suffering from atherosclerosis.

You must be able to develop the ability to mentally visualize the vascular system of your deconditioned heart. Then visualize the difference that conditioning makes. Think about the difference in blood and oxygen supply to your heart.

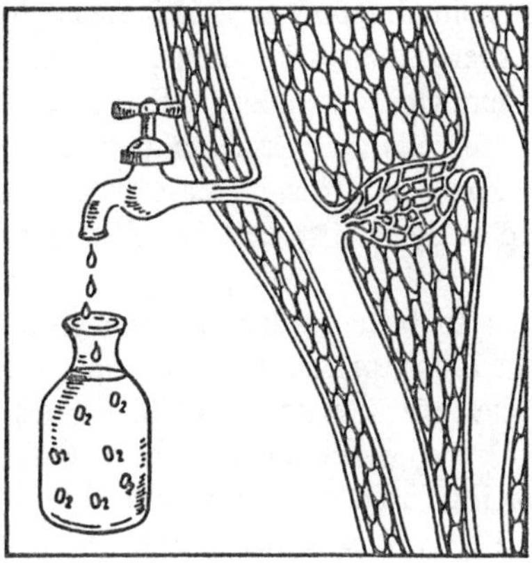

Expanded blood volume: Conditioned blood expands in volume and results in increased hemoglobin and oxygen delivery to body cells.

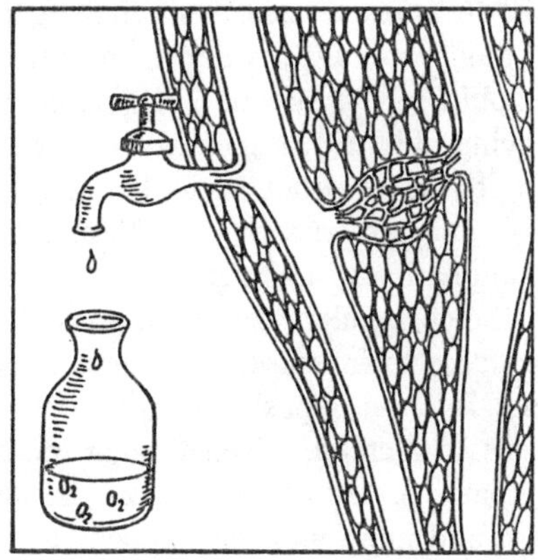

Deconditioned blood: Normal blood volume with no improvement in oxygen availability.

The Blood and Blood Vessels

Regular, sustained exercise seems to have profound effects on the blood and blood vessels.

In regard to the blood itself, the volume may increase up to one quart

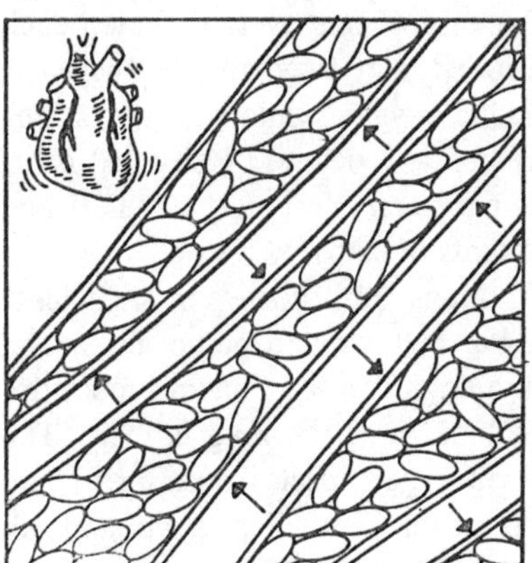

Conditioned arteries: Regular, sustained exercise causes an increase in the elasticity of the arteries so that the blood pressure goes down.

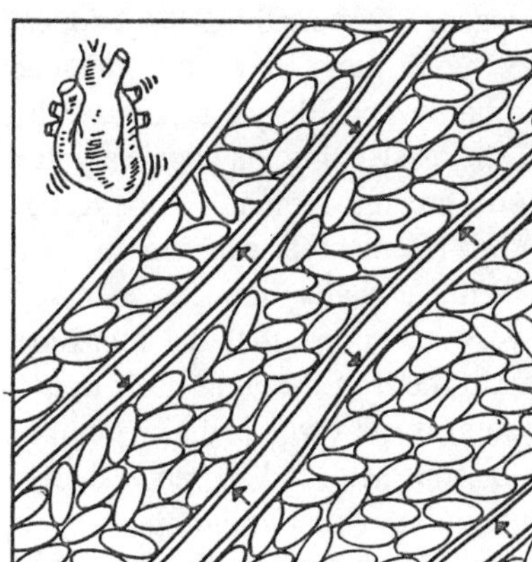

Deconditioned arteries: The arteries become rigid. With a loss of elasticity the blood pressure goes up.

in an average-sized man with regular, sustained exercise. This increase in blood volume provides a proportionate increase in the amount of hemoglobin in the blood. This increase in hemoglobin results in the blood's being able to transport more oxygen to the cells and tissues and to carry more waste products to the lungs for expulsion. This increase in blood volume provides the spark for increased body energy and more efficient elimination of waste products.

Since regular exercise causes the heart to beat harder and the blood volume to increase, you might think that blood pressure will go up. Not so. Just the opposite happens. Exercise causes the elasticity of blood vessels to increase. Even though the blood may be leaving the heart under greater pressure, the vessels—because of increased elasticity—are able to expand more and this explains why those who have hypertension and exercise regularly usually experience a fall in blood pressure.

What you must do is develop the ability to visualize this increase in blood volume and hemoglobin. Picture your blood vessels as they become more elastic—better able to expand as the heart contracts. Get a mental picture of this happening and your blood pressure returning to or remaining normal.

The Lungs

The lungs are magnificently efficient and delicate organs which are designed to deliver oxygen to the blood and remove waste material from the blood. The lungs are designed so they can provide sufficient oxygen in order that every cell of the body is provided with maximum amounts of oxygen. But something has happened. Because of our overautomated society, your lungs have become deconditioned and lazy. While they can probably provide your body with sufficient oxygen while you are sitting down or sleeping, as soon as you experience any degree of physical exertion (greater demand for oxygen) what happens? You start to "huff and puff." (Remember running up the three flights of steps?)

What actually happens to cause your lungs to become so inefficient? Everyone knows that the lungs are like big bellows and pump air in and out. True, but the lung itself does no pumping. The lung has no muscular system of its own. From a pumping point of view, the lung is inert. The lung contracts and expands due to the rib cage muscles pushing in and out and the diaphragm pushing up and down. The diaphragm and rib cage muscles are just like the heart and all other muscles; lack of activity and lack of exercise results in loss of strength and effectiveness. Since the contraction and expansion of the lung is based upon the activity of these muscles, inactivity will cause the lung to function at only a fraction of its capacity.

How do we measure the effectiveness of the lungs? Lung function can be measured by a test called vital capacity. It works like this. When you exhale, it is obvious you do not expend all the air in the lungs. If you did, the lungs would collapse. Usually 25 percent of the air is retained. Vital capacity is that amount of air you expel, still leaving your reserve in the lungs. This is the working capacity of the lungs. This working capacity (vital capacity) may not differ greatly between the conditioned and the deconditioned lung. However, a big difference can be noted when both have vital capacity measured during exercise. Because of superior development of the rib cage muscles and the diaphragm, the conditioned person can, over a measured period of time, inhale and exhale twice the amount of air. This results in delivery of twice as much oxygen to the body and the expulsion of twice as much waste products.

How do you exercise the rib cage muscles and the diaphragm? How do you make them stronger? By breathing deeply over a long period of time. How is this accomplished? Through regular, sustained exercise. Many people tell me as they begin their exercise program that one of the first places they notice muscle soreness is in the rib cage. This is great! Your tired and lazy lung pumping muscles are starting to wake—they are starting to come alive. Soon your lungs will begin to behave like the conditioned organs they should be. You will be supplying maximum amounts of oxygen to all parts of the body and getting rid of maximum amounts of waste products.

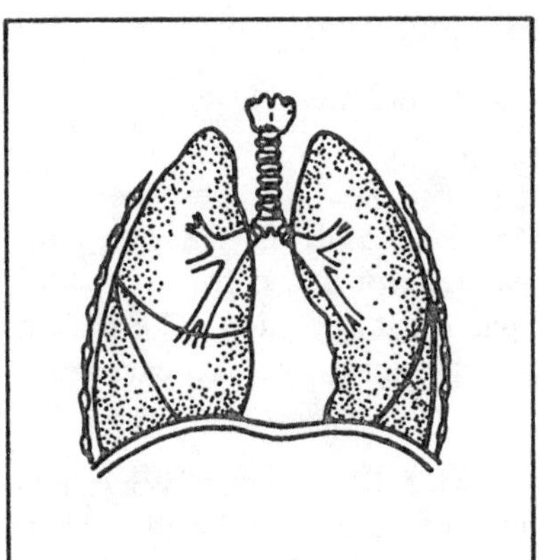

Conditioned lungs: The diaphragm and rib cage muscles are firm and strong. All lobes of the lung are operational, with maximum oxygen–carbon dioxide exchange.

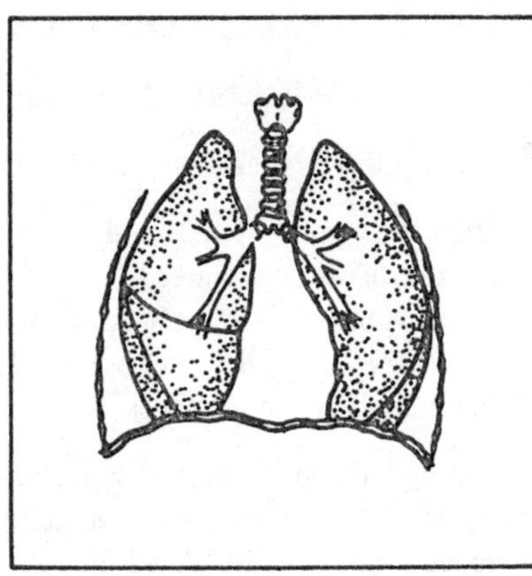

Deconditioned lungs: The diaphragm and rib cage muscles are weak and flimsy. The lower lobes of the lung are underused. The oxygen–carbon dioxide exchange is minimal.

Illustrated on the right on page 209 are deconditioned lungs. Illustrated on the left are well-conditioned lungs. Notice the difference in the integrity of the lower portion of the lungs. You must develop the ability to mentally visualize your deconditioned lungs, the lower portion ineffective, not able under any exertion to give maximum performance.

As you formulate your visualization program, you must be able to develop the picture of your deconditioned pulmonary system as it now exists, your rib cage muscles and diaphragm weak and lazy, not being able to contract and expand the lungs so as to work the lungs to full capacity. Visualize the lower lobes of the lungs going along for the ride, not really contributing to the delivery of oxygen or the removal of waste products. Next you must be able to envision your pulmonary system as it will be after it has reached a high level of conditioning. The rib cage muscles will be firm and tight, the diaphragm well developed. You must picture this entire muscle system contracting and relaxing all lobes of the lungs. Think about your pulmonary system being exercised and your conditioned lungs taking in twice as much air as they are now capable of processing.

Blood Chemistry

A number of studies have been published recently which report on the effect of regular, sustained exercise on blood chemistry. Blood chemistry refers to the various products of metabolism which are transported by the blood. Some of these which respond to exercise are: cholesterol, triglycerides, and high-density lipoproteins. This subject is considered in depth in chapter 6. However, a brief review and summation is in order here.

Regular, sustained exercise will cause the following:

Lowered cholesterol—a reduction in blood cholesterol levels.

Lowered triglycerides—a reduction blood triglycerides.

Increased high-density lipoprotein (HDL)—HDL is the so-called "cholesterol scavenger." It picks up cholesterol and carries it to the liver where it is metabolized and prepared for excretion. The higher the level of HDL, the better. Regular, sustained exercise causes an increase in your blood HDL.

Though there is some disagreement, the general consensus is that as the body is transformed from the deconditioned to the conditioned state, the favorable changes in blood chemistry are most dramatic. As exercise is increased from 20 to 30 minutes of continuous exercise to 45 to 60 continuous minutes, there will usually be additional improvement, though less pronounced.

From this it can be seen that a program of regular, sustained exercise has a well-defined positive effect on a wide spectrum of blood chemistry.

The Muscles

One of the most visible results of being deconditioned is flabby muscles. Muscles that are not exercised atrophy. They become soft and weak. At no place is this more evident than the lower abdomen, the "potbelly." This is an affliction which strikes men and women. Often the protruding tummy is the product of two segments of deconditioning. First, there are several layers of muscles over the lower abdomen which support the intestines and stomach. With deconditioning, these muscles become thin and weak and the pressure of the intestines and other internal organs pushing out is greater than the ability of these muscles to support. This is particularly true of a woman who has had a baby. In these cases, the protruding tummy becomes pronounced. Second, fat tissue has a tendency to collect around the middle part of the body. The collection of this extra tissue adds to the sagging nature of the "bay window."

Are you afflicted with the potbelly syndrome? It is a sure sign of deconditioning. It is not attractive and has a tendency to make a person, male or female, look older. The way to erase the problem is through regular, sustained exercise. Depending upon the correct selection of exercise programs, the muscles of the lower abdomen can quickly be conditioned, brought back to life, and made strong and firm. In addition, the exercise will utilize calories, which will remove the "inner tube" that has become inflated around the middle.

This example of the protruding tummy is only one of many I could use. It is presented because it is a problem that afflicts millions and because it is so visible. You can hide your deconditioned heart, lungs, blood vessels, and blood, but there is no way weak and sagging abdominal muscles and an extra twenty pounds of fat tissue can go undetected.

Why does muscle tissue respond and become stronger following an exercise program? Why are exercised muscles larger and firmer? Once again, the answer lies in blood flow. As you exercise (not isometrics), the individual muscle fibers become longer and additional routes for blood circulation are developed. The bulging of the muscle—the actual firmness—is caused by the accumulation of blood via these new and increased blood channels and growth of individual muscle fibers. With the delivery of this additional blood supply comes a super supply of oxygen from your conditioned heart and lungs. This results in additional energy and cell reproduction and growth at the muscle tissue level. This is why a conditioned musculature system always results in your having far more body energy. This increased energy leads to increased ambition, productivity, self-esteem, and self-satisfaction.

As you proceed into your conditioning program, the development of your musculature system is perhaps your first physical sign that "it's working." As your waistline starts to become smaller, your legs become stronger, your shoulders become less stooped, you will see in the mirror the end results of a conditioned body.

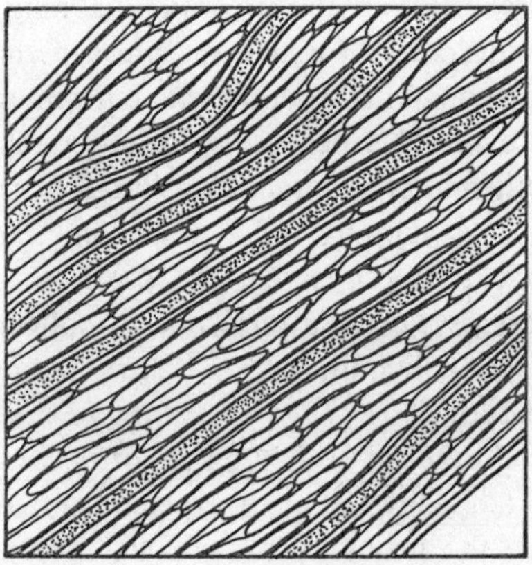

Conditioned muscle: The muscle fibers become longer and thinner, and the blood supply increases to maximum.

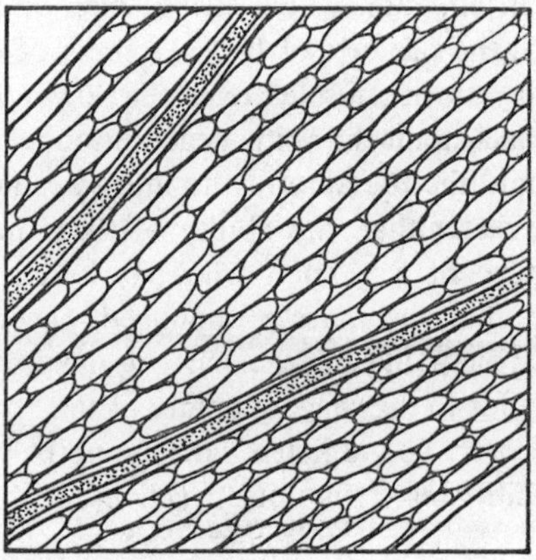

Deconditioned muscle: The muscle fibers are short and round and get minimum blood supply.

On the right is a cross section of deconditioned muscle tissue with a minimal blood flow supply. On the left is an artist's concept of well-conditioned muscle tissue. Notice the longer individual muscle fibers and the enhanced development of circulatory vessels.

Develop a mental picture of what lazy, soft, blood-malnourished muscle tissue looks like; then contrast in your mind the long, slim, sleek, blood-enlarged muscle fibers that make up conditioned muscles. Premature aging is easy to see in your deconditioned muscle system. Turn it around. A comprehensive program for physical fitness is the solution for your sagging body.

Body-wide Positive Effects of Conditioning

Several other organs and body systems are devastated by deconditioning and can be corrected by conditioning. The digestive tract becomes inefficient with deconditioning. Gastric acids oversecrete and the muscles of the large bowel become lazy. Conditioning has a calming effect on the hassle of the everyday world and slows down gastric acid secretion. The muscle tone of the bowel increases so that bowel movements are regular.

Exercise is the world's best tranquilizer and laxative. In chapter 5, the psychological impact of exercise is considered in depth, along with how exercise relates to stress, sleep, and behavioral response to diseases. Even though you may not have a problem with stress and worry, I suggest you read chapter 5 and learn how physical conditioning has a tremendous impact on mental conditioning.

There are numerous other body-wide positive effects of conditioning. I have covered the primary organs and body systems that benefit and have tried to inform you how and why conditioning is good. Let's turn now from a consideration of the effects of deconditioning and conditioning to the physiology of exercising and how and why exercising is beneficial. We also want to cover how much and what kind of exercise.

BUILDING YOUR EXERCISE PROGRAM

I have studied carefully the exercise phenomenon that started in this country in the early and mid-1970s. Many people and factors were involved in causing this unexpected event, but certainly one of the most influential was Dr. Kenneth H. Cooper. Dr. Cooper had a book published in 1968 entitled *Aerobics* (New York: M. Evans & Company). It was one of the first publications to clearly define a system for placing certain values (points) on various exercises. It was the first time someone told us: "If you want to be in top physical condition, here is what you must do." All of us in the wellness movement owe a debt of thanks to Dr. Cooper for making us aware of the value of physical fitness and showing us a way to achieve it. I can recommend the reading of this and other books on aerobics that Dr. Cooper has written.

Exercises are basically divided into four categories. They are:

Isometrics
Isotonics
Anaerobics
Aerobics

Isometrics

This exercise is performed by contracting a muscle or muscle group against an immovable object. Ten years ago, isometrics was the thing to do. The claim is that it increases muscle size and strength with minimal effort. A number of serious athletes jumped on the isometric bandwagon. Today few use this type of muscle development exercise. The problem with isometrics is that it causes a shortening of the muscle fibers and does not develop new blood supply routes. Sustained, movement-type exercise does just the opposite. It lengthens muscle fibers and results in additional blood supply.

Isometrics does nothing to improve the function of the heart or lungs. In fact, it may be harmful. Isometrics creates a significant increase in body oxygen demand. The only way the body can be provided this extra supply of oxygen is for the heart to work harder. As the heart works harder, the heart muscle itself must have more oxygen. If the lungs are deconditioned (which they are if isometrics is the only form of conditioning), sufficient quantities of oxygen cannot be provided for the oxygen-starved heart. The results in the coronary-prone individual could be a heart attack. Several studies have suggested that blood pressure goes up significantly during isometric exercising.

So, in summary, isometrics is effective in building muscle size and perhaps strength. The effect it has in shortening muscle fibers and the zero effect it has on cardiopulmonary development causes it to be a program that cannot be recommended.

Isotonics

This is exercise in which muscles are contracted and movement is involved. The best example would be calisthenics. In calisthenics you are stretching, contracting, pulling and pushing muscles. Other activities fall into this category: golfing (not riding a cart), bowling, heavy gardening, weight lifting, etc. Calisthenics is good in that it lengthens muscle fibers and may cause a modest improvement in blood flow. Muscle definition and strength will improve. The big problem with calisthenics is that, like isometrics, it does little or nothing to condition the heart and lungs.

Isotonic exercises do little for the development of the rib cage muscles and diaphragm. They do not cause the heart rate to be maintained at high levels for sustained periods of time. In short, while isotonic exercises will do you no harm, they do little to enhance your cardiopulmonary efficiency. They do little to increase your body's ability to consume and utilize more oxygen. In spite of this, I am a firm believer in calisthenics—calisthenics in conjunction with aerobic (best for heart and lungs) exercises. I will elaborate on this later.

Since weight lifting is an isotonic exercise, a special word must be directed toward this activity. When considering weight lifting, it is important to distinguish between those who are lifting light weight on a universal-type exercise machine and those who are serious heavyweight lifters. The former should probably not be considered a weight lifter in the strict sense of the word. When I refer to weight lifter, I am referring to the heavy-weights—those who are attempting massive muscle development. First, the literature points out that the majority of weight lifters have high blood pressure. Second, weight lifting (like isometrics) does nothing to improve the function of the lungs and heart. Third, it has been suggested weight lifters have a tendency to gain weight when their weight-lifting days are over.

I know a number of weight lifters. They are dedicated and I have been around long enough to know my comments will do little to dissuade them. For this reason, I do not suggest that anyone give up weight lifting. What I recommend is to supplement your weight lifting with an exercise program that will develop your heart and lungs as you develop your biceps and deltoids and lower your blood pressure as you increase caloric utilization. What is suggested is a program of aerobic exercise along with the weight lifting. Before discussing aerobic exercise, let's define *anaerobic* exercise.

Anaerobic Exercise

This means "without oxygen." This exercise is so intense and vigorous that the body demand for oxygen is greater than the lungs and heart can supply. If you are deconditioned and go out to the high school track and start running as fast as you can, the oxygen demand by the body quickly exceeds that which can be delivered. Even though you are breathing as deeply and rapidly as possible, you still cannot bring enough oxygen. You must either stop or slow down the running in order to reduce oxygen demand. If you don't, you will probably pass out.

There are also less vigorous anaerobic exercises such as riding a bicycle at high speed for short distances or swimming all out for several laps. These activities produce definite and major oxygen deficits. Due to the fact these exercises cannot be sustained, they are useless in regard to increasing cardiopulmonary efficiency and could be dangerous, even in the conditioned individual.

Aerobic Exercise

This means "with oxygen." It is any exercise that is done with enthusiasm, yet the oxygen demand of the body is satisfied. Thus, the exercise can be continued for extended periods of time.

Aerobic exercise can best be explained as follows: the deconditioned body starts an exercise program with the level of intensity that can be sustained for five minutes (this may be a jogging-walking program, swimming-floating program, riding a bike, etc.). With the passing of time and regular and increasing exercise periods, the body demands more oxygen. This demand is met due to the gradual conditioning that is occurring to the heart and lungs. Slowly but steadily the heart gets stronger and starts to pump more blood with each contraction. Slowly but steadily the muscles of the rib cage and the diaphragm become stronger so that the lungs can process more oxygen-rich air and waste products. This means that a greater amount of oxygen is available to the blood and more carbon dioxide can be exhaled.

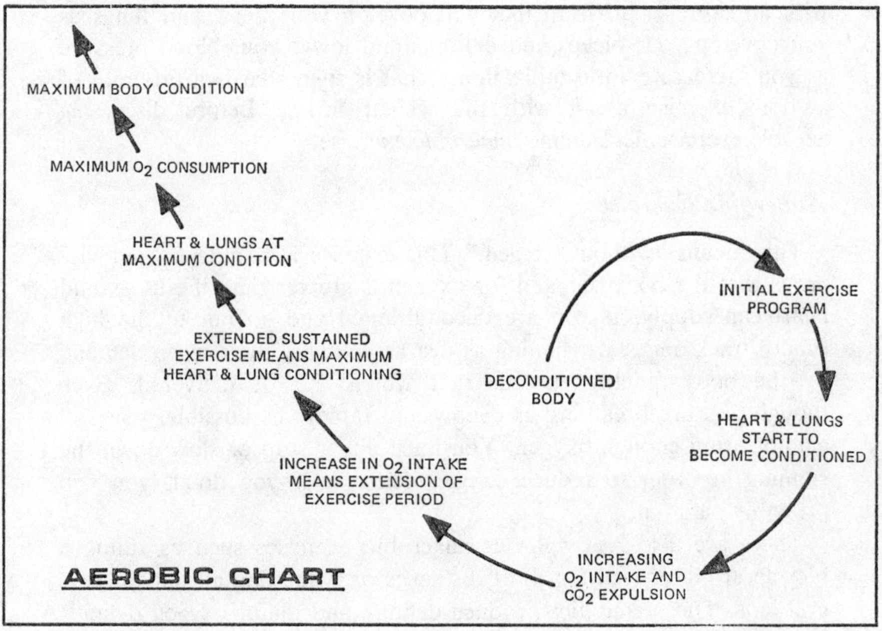

I use this chart when conducting Wellness Seminars to illustrate what aerobic exercising is all about. The chart may look complicated, but it isn't. Remember, when thinking of your deconditioned state, you must think not of your body being deconditioned, but of your individual organs being deconditionted. Think of your heart as being tired and lazy. Your lungs can process only one half the amount of air they should. Initially, aerobic exercising evolves around the heart and lungs.

As you can see from the chart, the deconditioned body, lungs, and heart are started on a slow program of regular and sustained exercise (we will cover how much in the section on heart rate). Slowly the heart and lungs start to wake up and respond to this extra exertion.

They respond by becoming stronger and more efficient. This results in increased amounts of oxygen being available and delivered throughout the body. This increased oxygen supply means increased energy. Increased energy allows the periods of exercise to extend. This constantly increasing exercise continues heart and lung conditioning until they are at maximum conditioning. At this point, the body is being delivered the maximum level of oxygen. Now you are where you want to be. MAXIMUM OXYGEN CONSUMPTION. You have arrived at that point of heart and lung conditioning where they are operating at maximum efficiency. The body is now being provided with sufficient oxygen so that you are exercising at your maximum speed and duration. You are in top physical condition.

Dr. Cooper has calculated the following oxygen consumption chart based on jogging one mile.

If you cover one mile in:	*Your oxygen consumption is:*
17.5 minutes	7 ml/kg/minute
13.0 minutes	14 ml/kg/minute
11.0 minutes	21 ml/kg/minute
9.0 minutes	28 ml/kg/minute
7.0 minutes	35 ml/kg/minute
under 6.5 minutes	42 ml/kg/minute

I have taken the liberty of using an average time instead of a time spread. It is from this information that the aerobic point system grew. The point I want to make is this. If it now takes you 13 minutes to cover a mile—this is a fast walk or very slow jog—and you want to improve to a 9-minute mile—which is an average easy jog for most people—you must *double* your oxygen consumption. You must condition your heart and lungs until they are able to deliver twice the amount of oxygen they are now capable of delivering. If you want to cover a mile in under 6.5 minutes (now you are running!), your heart and lungs must deliver *3 times* more oxygen. They must triple in efficiency!

I trust you now understand the importance of aerobic exercise to physical fitness. It doesn't matter if it now takes you 17.5 minutes to cover a mile—you can improve. The degree of individual improvement depends on a number of factors. When you can accomplish a 6.5-minute mile, you will have definite proof that your heart and lungs are functioning at a level *seven times* more efficiently than when you started on your way to high-level fitness and high-level wellness.

I find this is one of the most effective pieces of information I have to convince people that they should begin today to convert their deconditioned heart and lungs to the efficient and smooth working organs they should be. I have been told by hundreds of persons to whom I have presented this material that for the first time they really understand what being deconditioned means. They now have an understandable scale which allows them to mentally visualize how and why oxygen consumption increases and how and why heart and lung function improves.

What Kind and How Much?

Two questions that I receive constantly are: "What are the best aerobic exercises?" and "How much should I initially exercise?" Let's take the first one.

I cannot advise you as to the best aerobic exercises. Only you can decide that. I can provide you with a list of aerobic exercises in order of their ability to develop oxygen consumption. Each of the following aerobic exercises creates oxygen consumption of approximately 31.5 mls/kilogram of body weight per minute and are approximately equal in oxygen consumption. In other words, one 8-minute mile of running is equal to 12.5 minutes of medium-fast running-in-place, is equal to swimming 600 yards in 15 minutes, etc.

EXERCISE	DURATION
Running	1 mile in less than 8 minutes
Stationary run. 650 steps/min.	12.5 minutes
Swimming	600 yards in less than 15 minutes
Cycling	5 miles in less than 20 minutes
Handball	35 minutes
Walk	2.5 miles in less than 33 minutes

Other exercises could be added to the list, such as rowing, jumping rope, and golf (if you walk and carry your own bag). Any exercise will do as long as it can be sustained for a period of time without stopping. You need not confine yourself to a single exercise. The reason the above information is provided is to illustrate for you that they can be interchanged.

Personally I prefer a combination of running and calisthenics. I know my 30 miles per week of running conditions my heart, lungs, blood, blood vessels, blood chemistry, etc. In addition, certain muscles, particularly the leg muscles, are developed. Herein lies one of my complaints about running as the only form of exercise for physical fitness. Though running does have a tendency to firm up all body muscles, it often is not sufficient for the upper body. I am speaking of the upper chest, the shoulders and upper arms and forearms. As a matter of fact, if you notice the upper body development of those running considerable distances, it is usually thin. Since I feel that physical fitness should be directed to every vital organ and body system, this upper body thinness is unacceptable to me. This is the reason I prefer to do both an isotonic exercise (calisthenics) and the running.

I am not a supporter of lifting heavy weights, but I do suggest a one-hour workout on a universal-type machine several times a week. This is augmented with the good old-fashioned push-up, sit-up, body-bend type of exercise. I find this amount of isotonic exercise is sufficient to keep the upper body in step with my aerobic exercise program. The main point is that the calisthenics are done in addition to the running and never detracts from it.

Now that you are knowledgeable about the kind of exercising you should be doing, the next question is "How much?" I am assuming you are in an advanced state of decondition—haven't exercised on a regular basis for a considerable period of time—perhaps years. **The best initial advice I can give you is to check with your physician.** You will notice I did not suggest that you have an elaborate physical examination. Telephone or stop in and inform your physician that you would like to start on a preplanned exercise program. Let the physician determine if you do or do not need an examination. Follow the physician's recommendations.

As you start your exercise program, your main consideration is to go slowly during the first several weeks. You will probably find this difficult to do. After all these years, you are enthused, you have made the decision to never be deconditioned again, and here I am admonishing you to go slow when that's the last thing you want to do. After all, you have a lot to make up for. I am not trying to detract from your enthusiasm, but I want you to get started in the correct way.

If you have been sedentary for an extended period of time, your muscles, heart, and lungs are not accustomed to the exertion that your exercise will place upon them. You will notice that the oxygen demand of the body will quickly exceed the heart's and lungs' ability to deliver. Because of the lack of oxygen, you experience a buildup of lactic acid in the large muscle and this causes stiffness and soreness. You will "huff and puff" because of the inefficiency of the heart and lungs. Don't be concerned. I want you to know that these things will occur. Plan for them and don't be discouraged because you can't jog one lap without stopping or ride your bike for eight minutes without tiring. All of us who now run a number of miles started out just like you—not being able to make it around the track one time.

As you start your program, should you exercise to the point of exhaustion? No, definitely not. You should exercise according to your *heart rate.* In order to do this, we must first have an estimation of your Maximum Heart Rate (MHR). There are two ways to do this. If you want to determine your actual MHR, you must have a graduated exercise tolerance test, a GXT—called by some a stress test. This test is ordered by your physician and is conducted in the presence of a physician. You walk on a motorized treadmill while your heart, blood pressure, and perhaps respiration are being monitored. As the test proceeds, the speed and incline of the treadmill increases until your heart is beating at its maximum.

There is also a less complicated way. We now know enough about MHR's so that a formula has been developed by which you can estimate yours. This is referred to as the Estimated Maximum Heart Rate (EMHR). For men the EMHR is 220 minus your age; for women, 226 minus your age.

The monitoring of your heart rate during exercise tells you if you are exercising too much or too intensely. How do you monitor heart rate? By taking your pulse. There are two ways this can be done. You can use the radial artery, which is on the underside of each wrist, or the carotid artery which is on either side of the neck about one inch under the jawbone.

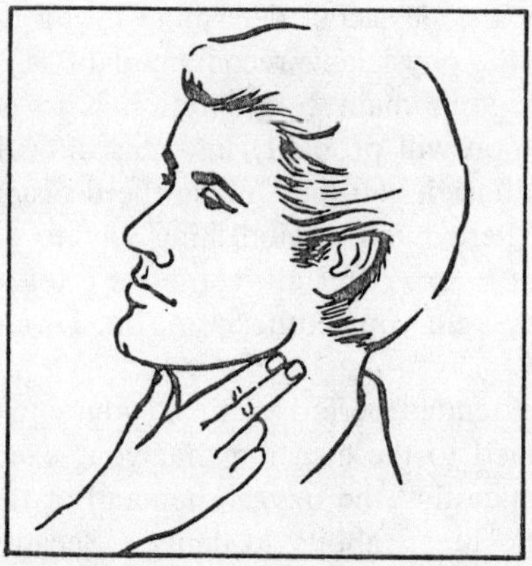

Carotid pulse

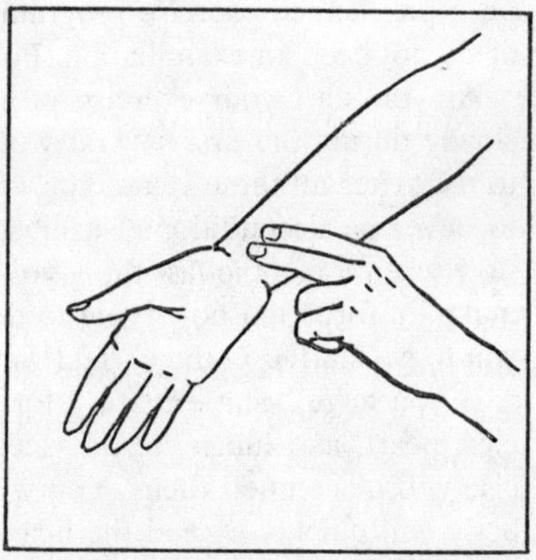

Radial pulse

The above illustration shows how to monitor heart rate. Most people use the pulsations of the carotid artery because it is the easiest to feel. One word of caution—don't press too hard because the carotid body is in this same area. If it is activated through palpation (pressure), it can alter heart rate.

As you start to condition your body, heart, and lungs, you want to be able to control your MHR. You don't want your oxygen deficit to become too great while conditioning is taking place. For this reason, you should follow the schedule below:

	MALE	FEMALE
	220	226
minus your age	________	________
equals	________	________
subtract resting HR	________	________
equals	________	________
1st and 2nd weeks		
multiply by .65	________	________
3rd and 4th weeks		
multiply by .75	________	________
5th week and thereafter		
multiply by .85	________	________
add resting HR	________	________
YOUR MAXIMUM EXERCISING HEART RATE (MEHR)	________	________

Conditioning Formula

In order to establish your Maximum Exercising Heart Rate (MEHR), take 220 or 226 and subtract your age. Then subtract your *resting* heart rate. As you start your physicial fitness program (first two weeks), multiply by .65. Then add your *resting* heart rate. This will give you your MEHR for the first two weeks of your program. At the end of two weeks, your heart and lungs have started to become conditioned, therefore you need to increase your heart rate during exercise. In order to do this, at the beginning of the third week calculate your MEHR by multiplying by .75. As you progress into the fifth week, multiply by .85. This will increase your MEHR to the maximum you should reach throughout your lifetime of high-level physical fitness.

It is realized that you cannot monitor or control your heart rate to each and every individual beat. You should adhere to your MEHR to the best of your ability. The main thing you want to do is not to exercise until you approach the MHR. Otherwise, it could be harmful.

As you become conditioned, you must be aware that both your resting heart rate and your MHR will probably decline. Once you reach top-level conditioning, your resting heart rate may decline 10 to 15 or more beats per minute. At the other end of the spectrum, your maximum heart rate may also decline. As I have already indicated, my resting heart rate is around 52. According to the formula, my EMHR should be 175. Yesterday my actual heart rate immediately following a brisk five-mile run was 125. For me, this is vivid evidence of the conditioning effect. My heart and lungs have improved their efficiency by over 27 percent.

Once you are past the five-week level, what should you have as a goal for exercise duration? How long should you run, walk, ride your bike, swim, play paddleball, or actually participate in your exercise? The answer is that you should exercise until you are pleasantly tired. Push yourself, but don't overexert. Listen carefully to your body. You will receive signals when you are overdoing it. I have been very fortunate in having run regularly for over nine years and never had an injury; however, I do get signals. If I run longer distances, say ten miles on consecutive days, on occasion my right knee will develop a mild pain. My knee joint is saying, "Careful, you might be overdoing it a little." I won't miss a day, but I will reduce the distance for the next day or two and the pain goes away.

While recognizing that there are individual differences in skill, endurance, desire, determination, and enthusiasm in each of us, I would like to suggest minimum goals you might wish to consider. After the five-week conditioning period, I find that most are striving for the following accomplishments:

EXERCISE	TIME
Running (8–9-minute mile)	30 minutes
Stationary running	30 minutes
Walking (brisk pace/nonstop)	45 minutes
Bicycling	30 minutes
Racquetball (actual playing time)	30 minutes
Swimming	15 minutes

These goals are not based upon research work, but upon the real world of what hundreds of people who have gone through the program are doing after the five-week conditioning program.

With the exception of racquetball, I find the average frequency of these exercises is nearly five times weekly.

These examples are provided as guidelines. You may want to exercise more or faster. Perhaps you will never reach this level. The main point is for you to push yourself until you bend slightly but don't break anything. There needs to be a modest amount of discomfort associated with your exercise routine, but don't go to the point where you are inflicting undue punishment on yourself. Physical fitness should be fun and enjoyed, yet somewhat demanding of your effort and time.

The Forgotten Muscles

What are the most forgotten and neglected of all muscles? Even for serious body builders, exercise enthusiasts, and the "young forever" set, there is one group of muscles that is almost always overlooked regardless of how comprehensive the exercise program. They are those muscles that reflect to other people your character, your age, your personality, your attitude, and your degree of physical fitness. The majority of our muscle systems are covered most of the time by clothing. Not so with this group. The condition of these muscles is open to public scrutiny all the time. They are the facial muscles.

The face is made up of dozens of muscles. These muscles are no different than any others. If they are not exercised, you have a deconditioned face. The facial muscles become soft, flabby, and lazy. With lack of exercise, the facial muscles age prematurely. To a great extent, sagging facial muscles are responsible for bags under the eyes, the double and triple chins, hanging jowls, excessive and loose skin under the chin, and the general relaxation of facial skin which contributes to premature wrinkling. All of these factors are enhanced if the individual happens to be obese. Deconditioned facial muscles cannot support the extra fat tissue and the sagging is exaggerated.

Self-image is a very critical part of high-level wellness. Your impression of *how* you appear to others is important. When interacting with other people, the face is almost always examined by the other party. Facial expression is one of the major methods of communication. For high-level wellness, it is imperative that your face be as young and attractive-looking as possible. The way this is accomplished is to include your face in your overall program of exercise and physical fitness. With the proper exercise program, you can firm up your face just as you firm up your midsection or upper arms or thighs. This firming up will reduce the incidence of baggy eyes, multichins, hanging jowls, and loose skin wrinkles.

How do you go about converting your neglected, deconditioned face to a firm, sag-free conditioned face? Through a series of exercises designed to allow you to be your own facial plastic surgeon. You may find that regular facial exercise as a part of your overall conditioning program can, in some cases, turn the sagging, tired-muscle face into the firm, skin-taut face you want to see smiling back at you when you look in the mirror.

Your facial exercise program must contain movements which will stretch and relax the major muscle groups. Following are several illustrations which show how they are to be done.

On page 224 on the left is an exercise designed to reduce the bags under your eyes and give you that "hollow cheek" look. On the right is one that will remove or reduce your multichins. They are only two of many facial

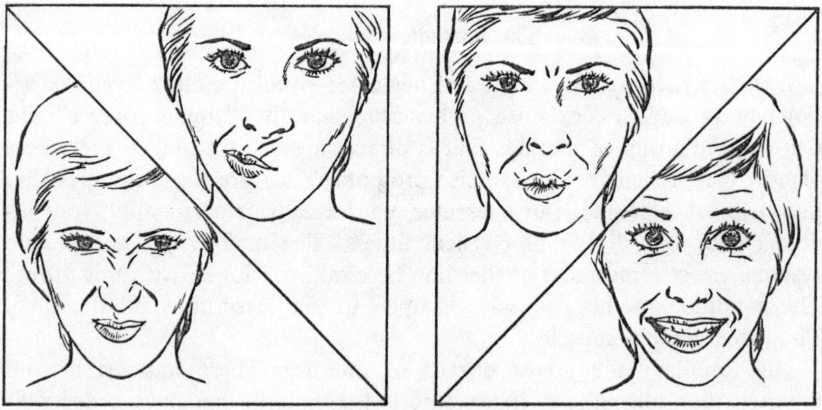

Facial Exercises

exercises you can perform. You can create your own. The main thing is to stretch and relax.

As you begin this face-conditioning program, your facial muscles will become tired very quickly. This is a sign of deconditioning. Don't overexercise. The main point is to increase the time devoted to each exercise. You should exercise until you can devote ten minutes each morning and evening to facial conditioning. You will be amazed how this twenty-minute investment per day can pay dividends.

Why People Fail

The major problem we have in this country regarding physical fitness is to get people to remain faithful and committed for a lifetime to a conditioned body, heart, lungs, blood, muscles, and face. I have heard the same story so often from dozens of people. "Yes, at one time I exercised regularly. I went to the YMCA four days a week, did twenty minutes of calisthenics, and jogged for two miles."

"Did you feel better when you were exercising on a regular basis?"

"Yes, I sure did."

"Well, why did you stop?"

"I really don't know. I slowly slipped from four visits a week to two, then none. Other commitments kept coming up which seemed important. I guess I just got bored with the exercise routine."

Let's stop for a moment and reflect on the types of exercise dropouts we have. First are those who start on a program and, within a month, before they have become conditioned, stop. The other group is made up of those who exercise to the point of top-level conditioning and then stop.

Why do weight lifters stop lifting weights? Why do swimmers stop swimming? Why do runners stop running? Why do calisthenics enthusiasts stop their routine? Why do bicycle riders allow the tires to go flat? Because of boredom, lack of excitement, lack of stimulation, and lack of motivation.

Let's be honest. For many, regular exercise is a bore. It does lack excitement and, in itself, does not provide much stimulation.

The main question, then, is: Why does this occur? It is because *the mind has not become conditioned!* The conditioning or development of the mind has been totally ignored. It is easy to understand why this has happened. Every exercise program ever developed has concentrated 100 percent effort on the physical aspects of conditioning to the total exclusion of mental conditioning. You are about to become involved in the first "total concept" mental-physical conditioning program. Just as you think of your heart, lungs, muscles, blood, blood vessels, and face as individual deconditioned entities into themselves, you must also think of your mind as being conditioned or deconditioned. How do you convert your deconditioned mind to a highly conditioned member of the team? By using your thought process and learning how to manifest the science of visualization.

Regardless of how many times you have started on an exercise program and not stayed with it, you are about to begin a program that will develop your mind and body to the peak of conditioning. You are about to become a member of that select group of people who realize that the way you treat the body does have a direct effect on how long you are going to live and the quality of life to be enjoyed. You are about to take direct control in determining your own health destiny and longevity. You are about to start a program that will cause you to feel better and live longer.

The key to remaining on a program of regular exercise is to totally immerse the mind in the subject of the harmful effects of lack of exercise, why and how it causes premature aging and premature death. At the present time, your body regulators are set to the reading that the sedentary life is okay. After all, it's the easiest way to live—no sweat, discomfort, or pain. Since the mind is ignorant of the devastating effects of lack of regular exercise, there is no reason for signals to be transmitted to the body demanding a continuous exercise program. Remember, the body can't think. It responds only to signals and direction from the brain.

So, the answer to the question "Why do most people abandon their exercise programs in one month or less?" is: lack of mind conditioning and education. Once the mind is educated, once it becomes convinced that the sedentary lifestyle is harmful, once it understands how and why lack of sustained and regular exercise destroys vital organs and body systems, once it comprehends that premature aging and death is caused by not getting sufficient exercise, an entirely different set of signals starts to be transmitted. These signals dictate to the body that exercise is a good activity and something that should be indulged in on a regular basis. When these pro-exercise signals are sent out, the body regulators readjust. Inactivity, the sedentary life, lack of exercise—these no longer have an okay status. The okay and required activity now becomes daily, sustained exercise. These changes in mind transmission do not happen overnight. It is a gradual change. The deeper and more in-depth the information provided for the mind, the greater the effort and determination to convert this information into knowledge and the faster the change.

You can *suspect* that the mind is becoming conditioned and starting to transmit pro-exercise signals when you start to look forward with anticipation to your daily exercise program. You can *know* it is happening when you feel guilty if you miss an exercise session. Much has been written lately about the "positive addiction" of regular, sustained exercise—particularly running. This is when a person actually may experience a type of withdrawal symptom if too many exercise sessions are missed. If you ever reach this stage, you can be doubly assured that your mind is totally conditioned and so well educated that very powerful pro-exercise signals are being sent to the body.

After the mind is educated, the conditioning program continues by providing visual before-and-after images of what the deconditioned organs and body systems look like now, and what they will look like after they become conditioned. Your mind, which after all does control the body, now has a well-defined target to shoot for. Now that the mind knows what is expected, signals to this effect are transmitted to the body.

Once you get your conditioned mind involved in your program, exercise will never be a bore, but an activity you look forward to. It will never be unexciting, but the highlight of your day. You will find that the internal lamp of stimulation is always lit, which will result in never-ending self-motivation. You will be at that point where you really are ready to accept your own responsibility for your regular, sustained exercise program, which is an important part of your overall program for high-level wellness.

The acceptance and involvement in a program for regular sustained exercise and physical fitness can be one of your most important efforts at high-level wellness. Before presenting your program which will result in lifelong physical fitness, I would like to summarize the overall benefits:

- Better cardiopulmonary efficiency
- Lower blood pressure
- Lower blood cholesterol and triglycerides
- Higher ratio of high-density lipoproteins (HDL)
- Increased coronary (heart muscle) circulation

- Reduction of excess body fat
- Increase in muscle size and strength
- Increased ability to consume oxygen

Can anyone be aware of the end result of regular, sustained exercise and not be anxious to start on a program immediately?

YOUR PROGRAM FOR PERPETUAL PHYSICAL FITNESS

Following is your personal program which will allow you to begin and remain on a program of physical fitness for the rest of your life.

Step One: *Make your personal commitment for permanent physical fitness.* You have already decided that elimination of the sedentary life is the negative lifestyle you most want to eliminate. If this is one of the first negative lifestyles you are going to cast aside, you have made a good choice because becoming physically fit often has direct or indirect positive impact on eliminating other negative lifestyles.

Now you must make your personal commitment. You already know that mind conditioning must take place before body conditioning. A part of this is for you to determine *why* becoming physically fit is important to you. Take time and identify the specific reasons. Perhaps it's so you can feel better, or so you can enjoy the comradeship that accompanies certain kinds of athletic activities, or so you can know the thrill of accomplishment. Next, you must decide *how* important high-level physical fitness is to you. Where does it fit in your other activity priorities? It should be at or near the top.

After you have given careful thought to these two questions and have answered them to your satisfaction, you should write a summary of your conclusions. Write in detail why this project is important to you and exactly how important it is. Your written summary communicates to your mind that you are serious about achieving mental and physical fitness and serves as a starting point for mind conditioning.

Concentrate all your mental and physical resources behind the elimination of this negative lifestyle. One of the greatest mistakes I see made is people with multinegative lifestyles become ultra-enthused and start on a program to eliminate all of them simultaneously. It won't work! Eliminating one negative lifestyle requires total concentration. I indicated that your mind must be conditioned, but the mind responds best if the challenge before it is singular.

Total, single channel concentration and effort will result in much faster and more permanent success.

So, regardless of how many other negative lifestyles you have, I want you to place all of your resources behind the elimination of your sedentary lifestyle and the permanent conversion of your deconditioned body, mind, vital organs, and body systems to a highly conditioned state. This will occur more quickly than you think. Then you will be able to move on to the elimination of your number two negative lifestyle.

Step Two: *Review and study again all the material in this chapter about how your sedentary life destroys vital organs and body systems.* You must read and reread the material in this chapter until you are comfortably and thoroughly informed about the effects of deconditioning on the heart, lungs, blood vessels, blood, muscles, and other body systems. Know the vital role oxygen plays in overall body function. Understand how and why deconditioning places a prohibition on oxygen delivery and waste expulsion.

Become an expert on exactly *why* and *how* deconditioning is one of the most prominent factors in causing premature aging and premature death. Learn how and why body, heart, lung, muscle, blood, and artery conditioning takes place. Become familiar with the various kinds of exercises. Understand maximum oxygen consumption. Learn the do's and don'ts of starting an exercise program. Know how to monitor yourself so as not to overexercise.

At the present time, your mind is without much-needed information and in itself deconditioned. You condition the mind by giving it information to assimilate, by feeding it with information as to how and why the sedentary life causes total body and organ premature aging.

Become your own information specialist. The more your mind knows about the devastating effects of the sedentary life, the more permanent will be your life of high-level physical fitness.

Step Three: *Develop the ability to mentally visualize your sedentary life destroying your vital organs and body systems.* There are numerous illustrations in this chapter. They are artists' concepts of what the deconditioned heart, lungs, blood vessels, blood, and muscles look like. As you are reading the material, study these illustrations carefully. Make sure you understand them and what they mean. Then you must commit them to memory. You must be able, on command, to visually create that same picture in your mind. Be sure you can visualize every minute detail.

Along with the deconditioned illustrations are companion artists' concepts of the same organs and systems in a highly conditioned state. The differences should be obvious. It is imperative that you have an accurate visual image of the conditioned state because this is the target you provide for your mind.

You must be able to play before your mental television the pictures of what you want your conditioned body organs and body systems to look like. You must be able to develop a mental picture of what is meant by maximum oxygen consumption. Visualize every cell in your body having a superabundant supply of oxygen for energy release and cell maintenance, growth and reproduction.

The two most important factors in your program are: first, providing the mind with in-depth knowledge about how and why the sedentary life causes premature aging and premature death; second, having the ability to visualize your body and organs as they now are and as they will become.

Step Four: *Write a summary of everything you learn.* It is a proved fact that your mental retention is better if you write new information down. For the majority of you, most of the information in this chapter is new. As you study the material, take notes. After you have finished the chapter and completely understand all the information, write your own summary. Write a mini-chapter of your own.

You can send mental messages as you think. This is good, but if you also send visual messages from the summary that *you* have written, you will more quickly accomplish your objective of conditioning your deconditioned mind.

As you are writing your summary, you should experiment with creating your own visualization illustrations. It isn't necessary for you to be a professional artist to draw meaningful diagrams of how the sedentary life is harmful to your vital organs and body systems. It doesn't matter if your illustrations are abstract. The important thing is for you to have a mental picture of the devastation caused by a life of little or no regular sustained exercise. Take the illustrations I have provided and improvise. Illustrations that you create will always be more meaningful to you. Remember that visualization must always include a before and after illustration. For this reason, be sure to produce drawings of what takes place as your individual organs and body become conditioned.

Step Five: *Establish and write down your goals for the accomplishment of your mental and physical fitness program.* The worst mistake you can make is to begin your program without reasonable goals. These goals must be measurable and well defined. The reason this must be done is so a constant increase in exercise effort is accomplished. The function of the mind is to be goal-seeking and goal-oriented. You will always accomplish more and in less time if definite goals are established.

Goal-setting is an important part of mind conditioning. It is a method whereby the mind can inform the body exactly what is expected. The body will usually respond if the objective is clear.

If you are a runner, a swimmer, a walker, or a bicycle rider, you should have a definite schedule of frequency and increasing time and/or distance. The same applies for any other aerobic exercise you choose. Until you are at the very top level of conditioning, you must continue to improve. This constant measurable improvement provides self-satisfaction, self-esteem, and pride, which are several of the factors that keep exercise from becoming a bore and every session exciting.

Once you have determined your goals, you must write them down. If you run on a track and your goal is to increase one or one half lap per week, write it down. If you want to increase your swimming by one lap per week, write it down. After you have established your goal and written it down, it becomes a part of the conditioning process for your mind. It becomes a command. Many people I know who are serious about lifelong conditioning keep a diary. Not only do they record their goals, but also their accomplishments.

Step Six: *Practice visualization techniques upon waking, noon, evening, just before going to sleep and while you are doing your exercises.* After you have all the required information about the technical aspect of your exercise program and have conditioned the mind along these lines, you are ready to begin your program of visualization. Just like having a definite schedule in performing the exercise itself, you must likewise have a definite schedule for visualization.

Your first visualization session is immediately upon awaking. You must develop the ability to visually picture in your mind all the harmful effects of deconditioning to your heart, lungs, muscles, blood, and blood vessels. Develop in your mental picture the details of how these organs and systems have become lazy. Next you should immediately picture what your organs and systems will look like after they have reached high-level conditioning.

During the day, it is best to relate your visualization practice sessions to your patterns of habits. Many people like to use routine occurrences such as the midmorning or midafternoon break at the office or some other such regular happening. It will only take a few days for the visualization session to become habit.

Visualize just before or after the noon and evening meals and just before falling asleep. The last visualization session of the day is probably the most important because the brain is very active during sleep. It can probably be conditioned better during sleep than any other time because the distractions of the day are absent.

Another ideal and "must" time for visualization is while you are actually exercising. I enjoy running on the open roads but sometimes run on a track. I often hear people comment on how boring it is running around a quarter-mile track again and again and again. The way to prevent this boredom is to condition the mind with your before and after visualization program. Regardless of your type of exercise, use the time to visualize. Use the time to condition the mind so the body will want to remain on your exercise program indefinitely.

Step Seven: *Develop a vivid mental image of you and your body in top physical condition accomplishing your predetermined goals.* It is necessary that from the beginning you develop the ability to visualize the finished product: an image of you, your heart, lungs, blood, blood vessels, muscles, and face all in top condition. Picture what they will look like after you have firmed up, lost weight, no longer have a protruding tummy. Try to actually *feel* what it is like to have your lungs processing two times more oxygen than now. Imagine your resting and MHR declining. Think what it will be like to have more than an adequate supply of oxygen delivered to each cell of your body.

Next you must visualize yourself already accomplishing the exercise goals you have established. If it is to walk one hour each day, picture yourself doing it. If it is to run in a 10,000-meter race, imagine you at the finish line at the front of the pack. If it's champion-level racquetball, visualize yourself receiving the trophy. Whatever your goal, visualize its happening and it is as good as done.

There you have it—your personal program for mental and physical conditioning which will last a lifetime. By launching your permanent program for top-level conditioning, you can be assured you are well on the way to preventing two of the worst human occurrences—premature aging and premature death. You are well on your way to high-level wellness and feeling better. You now have within your grasp PHYSICAL FITNESS TODAY, TOMORROW, AND FOREVER.

ADDITIONAL HELPFUL HINTS

At the end of each chapter you are provided with a brief outline of practical information, tips, and hints that are intended to supplement your visualization program. When used in conjunction with visualization, they will help you eliminate your negative lifestyle.

These helpful hints will aid you in achieving high-level physical conditioning in a safe and interesting way.

1) If you have been sedentary for a long period of time, it makes good sense to consult a physician before starting your exercise program.

2) Don't expect too much too soon. If you have been deconditioned for years, it will take time to reach the point of really enjoying your exercise program.

3) *Always set goals.* Physical fitness should be accomplished by ascending a series of plateaus. Initially, don't get stuck on a plateau. Increase your performance slowly according to a definite schedule.

4) *Have good equipment.* This does not necessarily mean the most expensive, but don't buy your running shoes, tennis racquet, or golf balls in the bargain basement.

5) Many forms of exercise are individual activities (jogging, walking, swimming, cycling). Though there are times when you need the solitude of individual exercising, don't let it become a habit. Enjoy the comradeship of exercising with others.

6) Establish a definite exercise schedule. Don't have the attitude that you will exercise when you have time. Set aside a definite time of the day and number of days each week you intend to exercise. Stick to your schedule. Soon it will become habit.

7) Don't confine your physical fitness program to a single activity. If you are a bicycle rider, learn how to play racquetball. If you are a walker, get on the tennis court and bat the ball around. You joggers might try riding a bike one day a week. This will help you develop different muscle systems and keep you from becoming bored and going stale.

8) Change your routine. If you are accustomed to running on the school track, try the roads or cross country. Ride your bike or take walks in different parts of town. Play tennis indoors and outdoors.

9) After you have reached top physical conditioning, enter competitive contests. Enter the local racquetball tournament. Run in the scheduled races. Play in the annual tennis or golf tournament. Don't be concerned that you might not do well. You will be surprised how well you will do. The competition brings out the best in you.

10) If you travel, don't let it be a reason not to exercise. Many cities publish maps of developed running, walking, and bicycling trails. Numerous hotels have affiliated with or can direct you to an athletic club or racquetball and tennis courts.

11) If for any reason you have been away from your regular exercise routine for one week or more, don't resume at the previous level of duration or intensity. Your heart can start to become deconditioned in several days, the body muscles in a week. Take a week or two to get back up to your previous level.

12) Don't eat immediately before or after extended exercise. A good rule is no food one hour before or two hours after exercising.

13) If you perspire freely during your exercise, replace the lost fluids by drinking small and frequent quantities of cool but not ice-cold water.

14) Some people like to go into the sauna or steam room after extended exercise. Be careful. Your blood vessels are already dilated from the exercise. The heat causes further dilation. This could be harmful.

15) There may be a fine line between procrastination and interpretation of the body's signals that you should slow down or not exercise on a given day. Develop the ability to distinguish between the two and take it easy when the body says you should.

16) If you wish, monitor your blood chemistry. Learn what your cholesterol, triglyceride, LDL, and HDL are. Determine if they improve as you convert from a deconditioned to a conditioned state.

10. YOUR FUTURE FULL OF WELLNESS

"The reality is in the dream!"
ROBERT H. SCHULLER

What is premature death? Technically, it's death prior to reaching the average age expectancy, which is around seventy-two years. The premature death that is most tragic is one that occurs at the age of forty-four or fifty-two or sixty-four. Have you ever answered the phone or had someone knock on your door and inform you, to your shock and surprise, that a close personal friend or close family member has died prematurely? Usually when a person dies prematurely, you ask, "Why?" Why did this person die at the prime of life or at the peak of a career? Even though the question is often asked, rarely does anyone try to find the answer.

If you pursue an answer, in many cases, you will discover that negative lifestyles have been a major contributing factor to premature death. Lung cancer, heart attack, stroke, liver disease—these and others can often be traced back to one or more negative lifestyles.

At the beginning of this book, we considered the Wellness Renaissance, which is starting to sweep across the country. People are beginning to realize that premature death is real, its causes are known, and it can be prevented. During the past several years, we have conducted considerable research to try and determine the overall awareness of wellness and the role one can play in determining one's individual health destiny. These data indicate that a typical bell curve exists. It looks like this: (See page 235.)

At one end of the curve are 16 percent of the population, who are already convinced of the value of assuming an active role in one's health future. They may or may not be familiar with the term "wellness" and the concepts of visualization, but they are well informed about risk factors and negative lifestyles. While most do not have a well-defined program

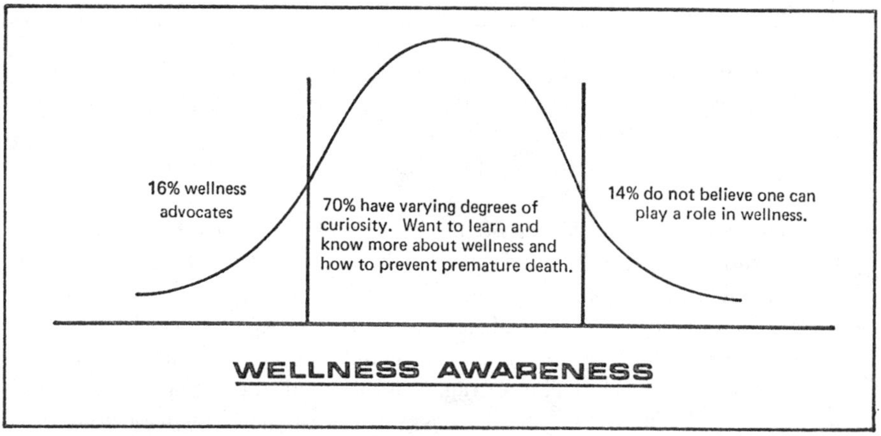

for the control of risk factors and negative lifestyles, they are taking some form of action.

On the other end of the spectrum is a slightly smaller group (14 percent) who are not knowledgeable about wellness and have no curiosity about it.

The largest group—approximately 70 percent—may or may not be familiar with the term "wellness" and its concepts and theories. Most are not actively involved in any organized program to alter lifestyle or reduce risk factors. Some believe that negative lifestyles are in some way harmful. Virtually all in this group are curious about their own health and want to learn more.

Where are you in this spectrum of wellness awareness? If you are in the first 16 percent, that's great. The programs contained in this book may be exactly what you are looking for. If you are at the other extreme—one of the 14 percent who are completely turned off by the idea that you can be instrumental in creating and activating your own plan to feel better and live longer—I hope you will reconsider.

If you are with the majority—one of the 70 percent who are curious about and ready to become involved in your own personal program for high-level wellness—I want to get you started by asking one question. If you were standing at death's door today, what would you give for another two, five, or ten years of a high-quality life? Think about it. You can't negotiate for these extra years once you have arrived at the time of death. However, you can start to acquire them today. The life of high-level wellness is the way to ensure that you will prevent premature death, feel better, and live longer.

IS THIS LIFE A BUMMER?

I have had an opportunity to meet a large number of people who are in the 70 percent group—those who have an open mind on the subject of wellness and want to learn more about it. In this group, even though they have a high degree of curiosity, there seems to be a universal initial reaction:

"Yeah, what you say about wellness preventing premature death, feeling better, and living longer sounds good, but . . . you are asking me to give up almost all the things I really enjoy in life."

Do you feel this way? Don't feel bad if you do, because, on the surface, to create a new lifestyle that does not include sitting at a bar and getting high and smoking seems like a drag. And, after all, how can you possibly find time every day for one hour to exercise? Just the thought of going on a diet and giving up many of the foods and drink you like is no way to enjoy life. All the complicated programs for stress control seem stressful in themselves.

People who have altered lifestyles and achieved high-level wellness are unanimous in their opinion that they don't miss the old negative lifestyles once they are gone. Some have said that the elimination of negative lifestyles leads to a greater appreciation for self-awareness. High-level wellness causes one to concentrate more time and energy on one's self instead of on the temporary pleasures that may be derived from negative lifestyles. This increased self-awareness results in a new kind of pleasure that is far superior to that obtained from excess alcohol, smoking, and overeating. Long distance runners have talked for years about the euphoria that results from sustained and regular exercise. It's real and it does exist.

What lies ahead for wellness as we know it today? What will happen as it matures and becomes full-grown? What will be the result of becoming more knowledgeable about premature aging and premature death? As we learn more about visualization and how it works, where will it fit into our everyday lives? The questions are limitless. Today as the Wellness Renaissance gains momentum, we are standing on the threshold of one of the most exciting breakthroughs of this century, the breakthrough that will allow you to play an aggressive, active role in determining your health destiny—how good you are going to feel and how long you are going to live.

What you have learned in this book is all you need to get you started on the road to high-level wellness. It will help you slow down the aging process. It can prevent premature death. With the passing of time, you will observe other developments in the area of wellness as the concept becomes better understood and gains universal acceptance. I would like briefly to review for you some of these future developments in the world of wellness.

THE WELLNESS CENTER

At the present time, a modest number of Wellness Centers are operating throughout the United States. By the end of this decade, Wellness Centers or Health Promotion Centers (they are the same) will be as numerous as hospitals or YMCA-YWCAs or health clubs or country clubs.

The Wellness Center is operated through a local hospital or by a private organization. Hospitals may be the logical operators of such a facility because they are community-oriented and are the experts in the delivery of services for the sick and the convalescents. Why should they not also become the experts for programs and services to keep the community well?

In many situations, the Wellness Center is an independently operated facility. Not being associated with a hospital does not detract from the Center in any way. Some of the best and oldest Wellness Centers in the country are privately owned.

A Wellness Center is not to be confused with a country club, athletic club, or health spa. *The Wellness Center is a medical facility.* It is operated under the supervision of a physician. Basically, a Wellness Center is a facility for education and behavioral modification. There are numerous other aspects which I will try to describe, but remember from the beginning the two major functions—education and behavior modification.

- The Wellness Center will provide continuous, ongoing educational and motivational programs to help people stay well. The programs are six to ten one-hour sessions on subjects such as stress reduction, obesity control, proper nutrition, accident prevention, smoking cessation, the theory of physical fitness, and elimination or reduction of alcohol and other drugs.

- There will be similar programs for individuals with various disease conditions. The goal is to help them better adjust to or cope with the disease. Classes offered may be on hypertension, diabetes, arthritis, selected types of cancer, and others.

- Individuals can go to the Wellness Center for comprehensive Computerized Illness Risk Factor Analysis. Physicians and other members of the health care team use computers to predict the percentage risk of a person developing certain diseases. Risk factors are identified, then educational classes are *prescribed* to help alter behavioral patterns and eliminate the controllable risk factors.

- The Wellness Center may offer facilities and programs for physical fitness along with exercise physiologists to *prescribe* medically sound exercise programs.
- Some Wellness Centers may provide live-in programs lasting fourteen to twenty-eight days. This total immersion concept may be the most effective way to alter behavioral patterns because you have the person's undivided attention twenty-four hours a day and there is constant reinforcement from others.

If there is a Wellness Center in your area, you should investigate and determine if it would be beneficial for you, but, I emphasize, *a Wellness Center is not necessary for you to achieve the highest levels of wellness.* Everything you need is contained in this book. Practice the programs as prescribed and you will learn how to eliminate all your negative lifestyles just as it is done at a Wellness Center.

WELLNESS AT THE WORKPLACE

The decade of the eighties is the decade for wellness to become a routine part of the corporate world. Companies both large and small have always been interested in the well-being of their employees. First, there was company-provided life insurance, then health insurance, then dental insurance, then optical insurance, all introduced to assist the employee with health-related problems. These will continue, but the corporate world is beginning to understand that prevention is far superior to cure and treatment. To this end, several large corporations started as long as ten years ago to provide company-sponsored physical fitness programs. Today this is common. In the 1980s, companies are providing in-company education programs that are designed to help employees at all levels to identify negative lifestyles and provide facilities and services to help eliminate them.

Companies are starting to install "high nutrition" lines in their cafeterias. A special serving line is available which features foods low in fat, cholesterol, sugar, and salt, and high in fiber and complex carbohydrates. On these serving lines, you find more fish, chicken, vegetables, fruits, and grain foods, and less red meat and desserts.

I know of companies that "pay for pounds." As an incentive, obese employees are paid a fixed fee per pound for weight lost. Others offer incentives for those who successfully stop smoking. Increasing numbers of companies are providing "stress buster" meditation rooms where employees can take a few relaxing minutes to get away from it all. Some offer cash for physical fitness activities such as jogging or swimming.

Many corporations are providing day-long Wellness Seminars for management and nonmanagement personnel. These Seminars are for most, their first introduction to the wellness concept and visualization techniques. For many it is the green flag as they start their race for wellness. It is the spark of stimulation which may lead to the self-motivation many need to become involved in high-level wellness. I have personally conducted several hundred such Seminars for the largest corporations in America. It is always a pleasure to interact with individuals and observe firsthand the intense interest they have in becoming involved in shaping their own health destiny.

Why are large corporations investing millions of dollars of profits and allowing employees to take company-paid time to become involved in wellness activities such as I have just described?

The corporate world has always realized the economic burden of absenteeism, illness, and unexpected employee death. Business is no longer content to sit back and allow these things to happen. Now that it is well understood that premature aging, premature death, and illness can be prevented or postponed, the 1980s and 1990s will be times of change as corporations help employees take control of their health destiny.

In summary, wellness at the workplace is for real. Wellness programs designed to keep employees well and on the job, well and feeling better, well and more ambitious and productive, will become a major *job benefit* and *employee assistance program.*

WELLNESS IN THE SCHOOLS

When considering all the potential applications of wellness during the decades of the 1980s and 1990s, none is more exciting or holds more promise for accomplishment than wellness in the schools. There are several reasons for this:

- Young people are more impressionable and flexible than the mature. They are better prepared to accept and try new ideas and concepts.
- It is far better and easier to educate a young person never to become involved with a negative lifestyle than to try to get an older person to eliminate one.
- If a person is convinced early in life never to become involved in a negative lifestyle, he or she avoids the potential devastating effects.

You might wonder if there is a proved need for wellness in the classroom. In a recent study by Dr. Stephanie Brown, it was pointed out that

30 to 50 percent of all nineteen-year-olds are moderate drinkers. Teenagers become alcoholics much faster than adults. Dr. Brown reports that it is not unusual for teenagers to be alcoholics six months after the first drink. Numerous reports have pointed out that alcohol is involved in the majority of teenage auto accidents. A study from Harvard University stated that 25 percent of children of smoking parents are themselves smoking regularly by the age of eight. The diet of the majority of our young people is a nutritionist's nightmare. One fourth of the boys and girls in grades 1 to 7 are obese. The main point is that we have created for the young people a society that is oriented toward premature aging and premature death.

During the next several decades, it will be realized by the appropriate agencies and organizations that instructing students on the merits of and how to achieve high-level wellness is just as important as reading, writing, and arithmetic.

Wellness for the youth of the country will be the single greatest step on the ladder of national wellness and the most important factor involved in increasing life-expectancy.

LIFE EXTENSION

Today's "Medical Futurists" are predicting life-spans of 100, 125, 150 years. Sound farfetched and impossible? Perhaps so, but the main point is that work is being done to determine *how* life extension can be accomplished. Just a few short years ago, all the funding, all the research, all the meticulous work required to convert theory to fact was being expended on treatment-cure procedures. Now increasing efforts are being directed toward dramatic, aggressive, and positive programs and methods for life extension.

As we look out into a future with a possible age expectancy of one hundred and over, what is being done to maintain mental youthfulness? After all, to expand the usefulness of the physical body and do nothing to improve mental acuity would be worthless. How do scientists suggest you keep the brain functioning at high-level performances for longer periods of time? Keep the brain active and stimulated. The brain circuits seem to change in direct response to stimulation from the environment. In animal studies, it has been found that if you raise rats in an unstimulating environment—plain cage with water and food twice a day—the cortex (gray matter of the brain) is of average density. If you take rats of the same strain, put them in a larger cage and add new toys every day and change feeding schedules, the cortex becomes 6 to 10 percent thicker. The brain that is challenged and stimulated develops more gray matter. Some have suggested that the brain responds like a muscle. The more you use it, the more it develops.

YOUR FUTURE

The future will be full of wellness. Yours begins today. You now have at your disposal everything you need to start your own life extension program. I cannot assure you that you will live to be one hundred or more years old, but I can assure you that premature aging and premature death can be minimized.

You now stand on the threshold of a new world. This is the world of mind-fitness–mind-conditioning. The programs that have been outlined for you are designed to help you educate and gain control of your mind's ability to send signals to your body. It is through mind-fitness–mind-conditioning that you visualize your way to the highest levels of wellness. Mind-fitness–mind-conditioning is not new, but so far only a select few have grasped its potential. Your visualization program is designed for you to bring into action the most potent power in the universe, your own thought processes. It is through this power that you will be able to achieve the ultimate goal in life—WELLNESS: FEELING BETTER AND LIVING LONGER.

Good Luck!